INDEPENDENT STUDY GUIDE

HIMSS CPHIMS 2026

Study Guide 2026

✓ Aligned to official exam objectives
✓ Adversarially verified practice questions
✓ Complete preparation resource

Meridian Certification Press
An imprint of Big Five Killer

HIMSS CPHIMS 2026
Study Guide 2026

Published by Meridian Certification Press
An imprint of Big Five Killer

ISBN 9798259502475 (Paperback)
ISBN 9798259502482 (Hardcover)

AI Disclosure. Portions of this book were drafted with the assistance of large language models. All content was reviewed, edited, and verified by the editorial team at Meridian Certification Press. Practice questions and answer explanations underwent adversarial accuracy review.

Accuracy Commitment. If you believe you have found an error, please report it to `meridian@bigfivekiller.online`.

First edition, May 2026.

Contents

How to Use This Guide

This study guide prepares candidates for the Certified Professional in Healthcare Information and Management Systems (CPHIMS) examination administered by the Healthcare Information and Management Systems Society (HIMSS). The CPHIMS credential validates the knowledge required to function effectively at a managerial or senior staff level in healthcare information and management systems. The exam consists of 115 multiple-choice questions delivered in a 120-minute (two-hour) computer-based testing window through Pearson VUE testing centers and Pearson VUE remote-proctored online delivery. Only 100 of those questions are scored; the remaining 15 are pre-test items used by HIMSS for future exam development and are indistinguishable from scored items. A scaled score of 600 (on a 400–800 scale) is required to pass. Candidates should verify the current testing window length and delivery options against the HIMSS Candidate Handbook in effect on the day they register.

The guide is organized into seven chapters that map directly to the seven CPHIMS examination domains in the 2022 Content Outline (still in force for 2026 administrations). The 2022 outline's domain weights — General 16%, Systems Analysis 17%, Systems Design 12%, Systems Selection/Implementation/Support/Maintenance 24%, Systems Privacy and Security 12%, Administration, Leadership, Management 12%, and Testing and Evaluation 7% — total 100% and are the proportions HIMSS uses to construct each form of the exam. Each chapter opens with the domain weight, learning objectives, and substantive narrative content, then closes with exam tips, key concepts, and five review questions modeled on the style and difficulty of actual exam items. After the chapters, a 50-question practice exam mirrors the proportional weighting of the real test so candidates can self-calibrate. Three appendices provide a quick-reference sheet, a glossary of 50 terms, and two ready-to-use study schedules.

The recommended study plan is eight weeks of structured preparation totaling 80–100 hours, or four weeks of intensive preparation totaling 60–80 hours for candidates with substantial recent experience. Either path follows the same sequence: read each chapter once for comprehension, take the chapter review questions cold, then return to weak topics for a focused second pass. Save the 50-question practice exam for the final week and treat it as a timed dress rehearsal. Score yourself by domain and review explanations for every item you miss as well as every item you guessed correctly.

Practice questions in this guide follow the HIMSS item-writing style: a stem written as a complete question or scenario, four lettered options, one unambiguously best answer, and three plausible distractors. Explanations cite the specific regulation, standard, or principle that supports the answer so candidates can extend their study beyond simple memorization. When a question references a regulation such as 45 CFR 164.312, study the underlying text — exam items frequently rephrase regulatory language and reward candidates who understand intent rather than wording.

On exam day, arrive at the Pearson VUE test center 30 minutes early with two forms of identification (one government-issued photo ID); candidates using OnVUE remote proctoring should complete the system check at least 24 hours in advance and follow Pearson VUE's environmental requirements for the testing space. Bring nothing else into the testing room or workspace; in-center lockers are provided, and remote candidates must clear their work surface. Pace yourself at roughly one minute per question, flagging difficult items for review and answering every question — there is no penalty for guessing. Use the on-screen calculator for any arithmetic; do not attempt mental math on workflow throughput, ROI, or sample-size calculations. Read each stem twice and identify the qualifier ("most likely," "best," "first," "least") before reading the options. If two options seem equally correct, look for the one that addresses the question's qualifier most directly. Trust your first instinct: change an answer only when you can articulate a specific reason the second choice is better.

The CPHIMS credential is valid for three years and renews through 45 continuing education contact hours documented in the HIMSS Learning Center, or by retaking the examination. Plan continuing education from the day you pass; it is far easier to log 15 hours per year than 45 in the final quarter of the cycle.

A note on agency naming. In 2024 the Office of the National Coordinator for Health Information Technology was elevated within HHS and renamed the Assistant Secretary for Technology Policy / Office of the National Coordinator for Health Information Technology (ASTP/ONC). This guide uses "ASTP/ONC" when referring to the post-2024 office and the older "ONC" when referring to actions taken before the renaming or when citing rules whose statutory text still uses "ONC" (for example, "the ONC Cures Act Final Rule" and "the ONC HTI-1 Final Rule"). Both names refer to the same office; candidates should expect either label on exam items and not be thrown by the variation.

General

Exam Weight: 16% (range 14–18%)

Learning Objectives: - Describe the structure of the US healthcare delivery system, including payer, provider, and regulatory actors, and contrast it with non-US delivery models the CPHIMS candidate may encounter. - Identify the principal federal regulations that shape healthcare IT investment and operations, including HIPAA, HITECH, the 21st Century Cures Act, the Information Blocking Rule, TEFCA, the ONC HTI-1 Final Rule and HTI-2 NPRM, and the CMS Interoperability and Prior Authorization rules. - Explain the major reimbursement models — fee-for-service, capitation, value-based purchasing, MIPS, alternative payment models — and how each shapes IT priorities. - Map common healthcare standards bodies (HL7, IHE, SNOMED International, LOINC, NCPDP, X12) to the data domains they govern, and describe USCDI as the floor data set referenced by certified Health IT. - Recognize the role of accreditation bodies (The Joint Commission, NCQA, URAC, DNV) in setting IT-relevant requirements. - Recognize 2026-current regulatory topics that are testable at the recognition level, including telehealth post-PHE rules, the FDA Predetermined Change Control Plan (PCCP) guidance for AI/ML SaMD, NIST Cybersecurity Framework 2.0, the CMS provider disincentives rule for information blocking, and patient-generated health data (PGHD) integration.

0.1 The US Healthcare Delivery System

The US healthcare system is the largest in the world by spend, accounting for approximately 17% of GDP in 2024, and the most fragmented among high-income nations. CPHIMS candidates must understand this fragmentation because almost every IT decision — from interface engine architecture to identity matching tolerance — flows from the absence of a single payer, a single patient identifier, and a single record locator. The system has three principal actor classes: payers (government programs and commercial insurers), providers (hospitals, physician groups, post-acute facilities, behavioral health, and ancillary services), and patients/members. Overlaid on this triad are regulators (CMS, ASTP/ONC, OCR, FDA, state agencies), standards bodies, accreditors, and the technology vendors who build, sell, and operate clinical and administrative systems.

Public payers dominate volume but not control. Medicare, administered by the Centers for Medicare and Medicaid Services (CMS), insures roughly 67 million Americans over 65 or with qualifying disabilities; Medicaid jointly funded by federal and state governments covers roughly 90 million low-income beneficiaries; the Veterans Health Administration, TRICARE, and the Indian Health Service round out the federal direct-care footprint. Commercial payers — UnitedHealth Group, Elevance Health, CVS Health/Aetna, Cigna, Humana — operate national networks under state insurance regulation. The ACA marketplaces and employer-sponsored insurance fill the working-age coverage gap. CPHIMS exam items frequently test the interaction between Medicare's Conditions of Participation, CMS Promoting Interoperability requirements, and a hospital's revenue cycle priorities.

Providers organize into integrated delivery networks (IDNs), academic medical centers, community hospitals, federally qualified health centers (FQHCs), critical access hospitals (CAHs), independent physician practices, and increasingly retail and virtual-first entrants. Each provider type carries distinct IT obligations. A CAH operates under a 25-bed cap and special cost-based reimbursement rules; its IT investments must prioritize interoperability with referral centers because case mix forces frequent transfers. An FQHC must report Uniform Data System (UDS) measures annually to HRSA, which drives population-health reporting design. An IDN must consolidate identities across acquired entities, making enterprise master patient index (EMPI) selection a board-level decision.

0.2 Federal Regulation of Healthcare IT

The Health Insurance Portability and Accountability Act of 1996 (HIPAA) is the foundation of US health information regulation, but the HITECH Act of 2009 created the modern federal incentive and penalty framework. HITECH allocated approximately $35 billion for the Meaningful Use program (now Promoting Interoperability) and substantially strengthened HIPAA enforcement. HITECH also extended HIPAA Security Rule applicability directly to business associates and introduced breach notification requirements.

Civil money penalties under HIPAA follow a four-tier structure that distinguishes the violator's culpability: Tier 1 (the violator did not know and could not reasonably have known of the violation), Tier 2 (reasonable cause and not willful neglect), Tier 3 (willful neglect corrected within 30 days), and Tier 4 (willful neglect not corrected). Each tier carries a per-violation minimum and maximum and a per-calendar-year cap for repeat violations of the same provision. HHS adjusts these amounts annually for inflation; the most recent formal inflation adjustment was published in the Federal Register in November 2024. As of that adjustment, the Tier 4 per-violation maximum and the per-year cap for repeat Tier 4 violations sit in the low millions of dollars, while Tier 1 maximums are substantially lower. Candidates should not memorize a single figure; instead memorize the four-tier structure, recognize that HHS updates the figures annually, and look up the current Federal Register figures during their final pre-exam review.

The 21st Century Cures Act of 2016 reshaped the regulatory landscape through three operational rules CPHIMS candidates must know cold. The ONC Cures Act Final Rule (45 CFR Part 170 and Part 171) implemented the Information Blocking provisions, which prohibit covered actors — health IT developers, health information networks/exchanges, and healthcare providers — from engaging in practices likely to interfere with the access, exchange, or use of electronic health information (EHI) except where one of eight defined exceptions applies. The eight exceptions are: Preventing Harm, Privacy, Security, Infeasibility, Health IT Performance, Content and Manner, Fees, and Licensing. Compliance dates phased in through 2022 with full EHI scope in effect since October 2022. The Information Blocking exceptions live at 45 CFR Part 171 Subpart B (exceptions that involve not fulfilling requests, §§171.201–.205) and Subpart C (exceptions that involve procedures for fulfilling requests, §§171.301–.303). The Security Exception specifically is codified at 45 CFR 171.203.

Information Blocking enforcement matured significantly in 2024. The OIG civil monetary penalty rule for health IT developers and health information networks/exchanges, finalized in mid-2023 and effective in September 2023, authorizes penalties of up to $1,000,000 per violation. The CMS provider disincentives rule, finalized in July 2024 (effective on a phased schedule across CMS programs), applies program-specific disincentives to providers found by the HHS Office of Inspector General to have committed information blocking — for example, loss of Promoting Interoperability category credit in MIPS, loss of MIPS Promoting Interoperability program credit for hospitals, and disqualification from the Medicare Shared Savings Program for an ACO that includes the provider. CPHIMS candidates should know that OIG investigates and refers; CMS applies the provider disincentives.

The CMS Interoperability and Patient Access Rule (45 CFR Parts 422, 431, 438, 457, 482, and 485) requires payers regulated by CMS to implement Patient Access, Provider Directory, and Payer-to-Payer APIs based on HL7 FHIR Release 4. The CMS Interoperability and Prior Authorization Final Rule finalized in January 2024 extends FHIR-based exchange to prior authorization workflows, including a Patient Access API extension to surface prior authorization decisions, a Provider Access API, a Payer-to-Payer FHIR API, and a Prior Authorization API based on the Da Vinci Prior Authorization Support and Coverage Requirements Discovery implementation guides. Compliance dates phase in through January 2027. CPHIMS candidates should know that the required FHIR base is R4 and that the US Core Implementation Guide defines the US-specific profiles.

The Trusted Exchange Framework and Common Agreement (TEFCA) became operational in 2023. ASTP/ONC contracts with The Sequoia Project as the Recognized Coordinating Entity (RCE), and it is the Sequoia Project in its RCE role that operationally designates and oversees Qualified Health Information Networks (QHINs). As of late 2025, Sequoia had designated a small cluster of production QHINs, with additional applicants in the pipeline. TEFCA establishes a nationwide network-of-networks supporting six Exchange Purposes as defined in the Common Agreement and the TEFCA Standard Operating Procedures: Treatment, Payment, Health Care Operations, Public Health, Government Benefits Determination, and Individual Access Services. The formal names matter on the exam: "Health Care Operations" (two words) and "Government Benefits Determination" (not just "Government Benefits") are the SOP-defined labels.

0.3 The ONC HTI-1 Final Rule and AI/ML in Certified Health IT

The ONC Health Data, Technology, and Interoperability: Certification Program Updates, Algorithm Transparency, and Information Sharing Final Rule — universally known as HTI-1 — was finalized in December 2023 and took effect on a phased schedule beginning in January 2024 (45 CFR Part 170). HTI-1 is a top-of-mind 2026 topic and is virtually certain to surface on the exam.

The HTI-1 Final Rule introduces three operationally significant changes to the ONC Health IT Certification Program. First, it updates the certification's data baseline from USCDI v1 to USCDI v3, with USCDI v4 anticipated as the next floor in subsequent rulemaking. Second, it introduces a new Decision Support Intervention (DSI) certification criterion at 45 CFR 170.315(b)(11) that replaces the prior Clinical Decision Support criterion and significantly expands governance expectations for predictive and AI/ML-based decision support. Third, it adds Insights Condition and Maintenance of Certification requirements that obligate certified developers to report a defined set of metrics to ASTP/ONC.

The DSI criterion distinguishes two classes of decision support: evidence-based DSI (rules driven by published clinical evidence or organizational policy) and predictive DSI (interventions whose output depends on a predictive model, including AI/ML models). For both classes, the certified product must enable the user to view source attribute information — the metadata that describes how the intervention was developed, what data it was trained on (for predictive DSI), what populations it was validated against, the intervention's intended use, and known limitations. For predictive DSI, the source attribute list is substantially longer and includes details about training data, validation populations, fairness measures, and ongoing monitoring practices.

HTI-1 also requires certified developers to support Intervention Risk Management Practices (IRMP). An IRMP is a documented practice covering analysis of potential risks and adverse effects of the intervention, risk mitigation, and ongoing monitoring of intervention performance after deployment. The developer must make a summary of its IRMP publicly available. Healthcare organizations that deploy DSI within certified products inherit operational obligations to use the source attribute disclosures, govern intervention performance, and adjust or retire interventions whose performance degrades. CPHIMS exam items in 2026 may test the candidate's recognition of source attribute disclosure, IRMP, and the distinction between evidence-based and predictive DSI.

The HTI-2 Notice of Proposed Rulemaking, published in August 2024, builds on HTI-1 and proposes substantial new certification criteria oriented to public health interoperability, payer interoperability, patient engagement, and additional API capabilities. As of late 2025, HTI-2 had not been finalized; candidates should track ASTP/ONC for the final rule and recognize HTI-2 at the proposal level. The MIPS Promoting Interoperability program for eligible clinicians and the Medicare Promoting Interoperability Program for hospitals are likely to import HTI-2 changes once finalized.

0.4 USCDI Versioning

The United States Core Data for Interoperability (USCDI) is ASTP/ONC's standardized set of data classes and data elements that certified Health IT must support. USCDI evolves through a public version process; the current floor for the Health IT Certification Program is USCDI v3 (incorporated through HTI-1). USCDI v4 was published in July 2023 and is anticipated to become the next certification floor through future rulemaking; USCDI v5 was published in July 2024 and is in the public iteration cycle. The USCDI process accepts public submissions of new data elements that progress through a Draft □ Level 2 □ Standard pathway based on use and maturity. CPHIMS candidates should know USCDI is the floor (not the ceiling) for certified Health IT and that USCDI Plus initiatives extend the base set for domain-specific use cases (cancer, quality, public health).

0.5 Reimbursement Models and Their IT Implications

Reimbursement model shapes IT priorities more directly than any other business factor. Fee-for-service reimbursement, still the dominant Medicare payment mode, requires accurate charge capture, complete documentation to support coding, and fast claims submission. The IT stack emphasizes computerized physician order entry (CPOE), clinical documentation improvement (CDI), and revenue cycle management. Value-based and risk-sharing models invert these priorities. Under the Medicare Shared Savings Program (MSSP), an Accountable Care Organization (ACO) bears risk on total cost of care for an attributed Medicare population and must invest heavily in population health analytics, care management workflows, and post-acute network coordination.

The Quality Payment Program (QPP) implements the Medicare Access and CHIP Reauthorization Act (MACRA) and has two tracks: the Merit-based Incentive Payment System (MIPS) and Advanced Alternative Payment Models (Advanced APMs). MIPS scores eligible clinicians across four performance categories — Quality, Cost, Improvement Activities, and Promoting Interoperability. Category weights are set annually in the QPP final rule. For the 2025 performance year, the published weights were Quality 30%, Cost 30%, Improvement Activities 15%, and Promoting Interoperability 25%; analogous weights are expected for the 2026 performance year, but CMS typically publishes the definitive CY 2026 QPP Final Rule in November 2025. **Candidates should verify the CY 2026 weights in the QPP Final Rule and on CMS QPP resources within 30 days of their exam date** and should not rely on memorized weights without confirmation. CPHIMS candidates should also expect questions on the linkage between EHR-supported quality measure reporting (CQM) and MIPS scoring, on the Promoting Interoperability category objectives, and on the CMS Health Equity Index introduced into the MIPS Quality category beginning with the 2024 performance year.

Bundled payment programs, including the Bundled Payments for Care Improvement Advanced (BPCI-Advanced) model and the mandatory Transforming Episode Accountability Model (TEAM) launching in 2026, package payment for a clinical episode (e.g., joint replacement) across the entire continuum. The IT requirements are post-acute data exchange, episode-cost attribution, and risk-adjusted benchmarks. The TEAM model is mandatory for hospitals in selected core-based statistical areas (CBSAs) for five major procedure categories.

0.6 Telehealth Post-PHE and Controlled Substance Prescribing

The COVID-19 public health emergency (PHE) ended on May 11, 2023, but several telehealth flexibilities have been extended by Congress or by regulators on a rolling basis. Three areas remain testable in 2026 because they directly affect IT design for virtual-care platforms.

First, Medicare telehealth flexibilities — the originating-site waivers, the eligible-practitioner expansions, the audio-only allowances for behavioral health, and the FQHC and RHC distant-site authorizations — have been extended through Congressional appropriations action. Candidates should expect questions on the operational status of CMS telehealth coverage and on the IT obligations (consent capture, place-of-service coding, modifier use) that flow from coverage.

Second, controlled substance prescribing under the Ryan Haight Online Pharmacy Consumer Protection Act of 2008 normally requires at least one in-person evaluation before a practitioner may prescribe a controlled substance. The DEA waived this requirement during the PHE and has extended the waiver multiple times through regulatory action. As of late 2025, the DEA continues to extend Schedule II–V prescribing flexibilities pending a permanent rule, and has proposed a Special Registration framework that would create a categorical telemedicine pathway with additional safeguards. CPHIMS candidates should recognize the Ryan Haight Act as the relevant statute, recognize that the in-person requirement is currently waived under a series of extensions, and recognize that a permanent rule has not been finalized at the time of writing.

Third, state licensure compacts — the Interstate Medical Licensure Compact, the Nurse Licensure Compact, the PSYPACT psychology compact, the PT Compact, and others — provide alternative licensure pathways that affect which providers may furnish virtual care across state lines. The compacts do not eliminate state licensure but provide an expedited pathway among participating states. IT systems for multi-state telehealth must verify provider eligibility under the applicable compact for each encounter.

0.7 Patient-Generated Health Data and Remote Patient Monitoring

Patient-generated health data (PGHD) — symptom logs, wearable readings, home blood pressure or glucose values, patient-reported outcome measures, and similar data captured outside a traditional clinical encounter — is an expanding category for both clinical care and reimbursement. Medicare reimburses remote physiologic monitoring (RPM, CPT 99453–99458) and remote therapeutic monitoring (RTM, CPT 98975–98981) under defined coverage conditions, including device qualification, minimum data days per month (commonly 16 of 30 days), and clinical review time. The IT obligations are device integration through FHIR or proprietary APIs, data reconciliation with the clinical chart, billing capture for the time and device codes, and a privacy and consent posture that addresses both HIPAA and state-level privacy law for connected-device data.

0.8 Healthcare Standards Bodies

Standards proliferation is one reason healthcare IT is hard. CPHIMS candidates should map each standard to its domain.

Standard	Steward	Domain
HL7 v2.x	Health Level Seven International	Real-time messaging (ADT, ORM, ORU)
HL7 CDA	HL7 International	Document exchange (CCD, Discharge Summary)
HL7 FHIR R4	HL7 International	API-based exchange, US Core profiles
IHE Profiles	Integrating the Healthcare Enterprise	Cross-vendor interoperability use cases
SNOMED CT	SNOMED International	Clinical terminology
LOINC	Regenstrief Institute	Lab observations, document type codes
RxNorm	National Library of Medicine	Medication terminology
ICD-10-CM	CDC/NCHS	Diagnosis coding (including SDOH Z codes)
ICD-10-PCS	CMS	Inpatient procedure coding
CPT	American Medical Association	Outpatient procedure coding
NCPDP SCRIPT	National Council for Prescription Drug Programs	E-prescribing
X12 5010	ASC X12	Claims and remittance (837, 835, 270/271, 276/277)
DICOM	NEMA/MITA	Medical imaging
USCDI v3 (with v4/v5 in pipeline)	ASTP/ONC	Floor data set for certified Health IT

The Da Vinci Project, an HL7 FHIR Accelerator, develops payer-provider FHIR implementation guides for use cases including coverage requirements discovery (CRD), documentation templates and rules (DTR), and prior authorization support (PAS). CPHIMS exam items in the 2026 cycle frequently reference Da Vinci IGs because they underpin the CMS Interoperability and Prior Authorization Final Rule.

0.9 Health Equity and SDOH Data

Health equity is now an explicit federal IT priority. USCDI v2 introduced a discrete set of SDOH (Social Determinants of Health) elements covering problems, observations, goals, interventions, and assessments; USCDI v3 expanded the set. The Gravity Project, an HL7 FHIR Accelerator, develops the SDOH implementation guides that operationalize these elements. ICD-10-CM Z codes (Z55–Z65) capture SDOH at the diagnosis level — for example, Z59.0 (homelessness) and Z59.41 (food insecurity). CMS has incorporated a Health Equity Index into the MIPS Quality category to reward eligible clinicians who deliver care to dual-eligible and low-income beneficiaries. CPHIMS exam items at the recognition level may test the relationships among USCDI SDOH, Z codes, and CMS payment program integration.

0.10 NIST Cybersecurity Framework 2.0

NIST released the Cybersecurity Framework 2.0 in February 2024 — the first major framework update since CSF 1.1 in 2018. CSF 2.0 adds a sixth Function — Govern — to the prior five Functions (Identify, Protect, Detect, Respond, Recover). The Govern Function captures cybersecurity governance practices including risk management strategy, supply chain risk management, roles and responsibilities, and policy. CSF 2.0 is widely used in healthcare as a complement to HIPAA Security Rule requirements: organizations map their HIPAA Security Rule controls to CSF Categories and Subcategories to demonstrate maturity beyond the regulatory minimum. NIST publishes a HIPAA Security Rule-to-CSF crosswalk that candidates may reference. CPHIMS items at the recognition level test the six Functions and the role of CSF as a complementary framework, not a HIPAA substitute.

0.11 Accreditation Bodies

The Joint Commission accredits roughly 80% of US hospitals and sets information management standards in chapters IM (Information Management), RC (Record of Care), and PI (Performance Improvement). Joint Commission survey tracers may follow a patient's record across systems; an interface failure that produces a discrepancy between the inpatient EHR and the radiology PACS becomes a survey finding. NCQA accredits health plans and certifies measures under HEDIS. URAC accredits a broader set of organizations including pharmacy benefit managers and telehealth providers. DNV is a CMS-deeming-authority accreditor used by approximately 15% of US hospitals and tightly integrates ISO 9001 quality management with CMS Conditions of Participation.

Exam Tip

When a question references a "covered actor" for information blocking, the three categories are health IT developers of certified health IT, health information networks/exchanges, and healthcare providers. Payers are not covered actors under the ONC rule — they fall under the separate CMS Interoperability Rule.

Exam Tip

The Information Blocking Rule has eight exceptions, but only the Content and Manner Exception lets a covered actor decline to provide EHI in a requested format if alternative manner conditions are met. Memorize the eight exceptions by category: two harm/risk-based (Preventing Harm, Security), two capacity-based (Infeasibility, Health IT Performance), three procedure-based (Content and Manner, Fees, Licensing), and one consent-based (Privacy). All eight live in 45 CFR Part 171.

Exam Tip

When a question references AI/ML decision support in a certified EHR, the relevant regulation is the ONC HTI-1 Final Rule and the relevant certification criterion is DSI at 45 CFR 170.315(b)(11). Key concepts: source attribute disclosure, evidence-based vs predictive DSI, and Intervention Risk Management Practices (IRMP).

Key Concept

US healthcare is a fragmented payer-provider-patient ecosystem; every IT decision must accommodate that fragmentation. There is no single national patient identifier and no single record locator service.

Key Concept

HITECH extended HIPAA Security Rule applicability directly to business associates and introduced criminal penalties enforced by DOJ for knowing violations. HIPAA civil penalties follow a four-tier structure adjusted annually for inflation.

Key Concept

TEFCA QHINs operate under a common trust framework administered by The Sequoia Project as the Recognized Coordinating Entity (RCE). The Common Agreement defines six Exchange Purposes including the formally named Health Care Operations and Government Benefits Determination.

Key Concept

Reimbursement model dictates IT priorities. Fee-for-service prioritizes charge capture and coding; value-based care prioritizes population analytics, care management, and post-acute coordination.

Key Concept

> The Joint Commission's IM chapter requires healthcare organizations to plan for the management of information across the continuum of care, which CPHIMS candidates should read as "your interface engine is a survey-relevant asset."

0.12 Chapter Review Questions

Q1. Which federal regulation directly prohibits practices that interfere with the access, exchange, or use of electronic health information by health IT developers, networks, and providers? A) HIPAA Privacy Rule B) ONC Cures Act Final Rule (45 CFR Part 171) C) CMS Interoperability and Patient Access Rule D) HITECH Breach Notification Rule **Answer: B** — The Information Blocking provisions are codified at 45 CFR Part 171 and were finalized in the ONC Cures Act Final Rule implementing the 21st Century Cures Act.

Q2. A hospital declines to share an electronic copy of a patient's record with a competing provider, citing security concerns. Under the Information Blocking Rule, which exception must the hospital document to defend this practice? A) Content and Manner Exception B) Fees Exception C) Security Exception D) Infeasibility Exception **Answer: C** — The Security Exception, codified at 45 CFR 171.203, permits a covered actor to engage in a practice likely to interfere with EHI access for security reasons if specific conditions are met, including a documented organizational security policy that is tailored to specific security risks and consistently and non-discriminatorily applied.

Q3. Which standard is the required base for the CMS Patient Access, Provider Directory, and Payer-to-Payer APIs? A) HL7 v2.5.1 B) HL7 CDA R2 C) HL7 FHIR Release 4 with US Core profiles D) X12 5010 **Answer: C** — The CMS Interoperability and Patient Access Rule and the subsequent CMS Interoperability and Prior Authorization Final Rule both require HL7 FHIR R4 with the US Core Implementation Guide as the technical baseline.

Q4. Under the ONC HTI-1 Final Rule, certified Health IT supporting predictive decision support interventions must enable users to view which class of information about the intervention? A) Vendor pricing and contract terms B) Source attribute information including training data, validation populations, and known limitations C) Patient-specific outcomes data D) Aggregate utilization statistics only **Answer: B** — The DSI certification criterion at 45 CFR 170.315(b)(11) requires that users be able to view source attribute information describing how the intervention was developed, what data it was trained on, what populations it was validated against, the intended use, and known limitations. For predictive DSI the list is substantially longer than for evidence-based DSI.

Q5. A critical access hospital is selecting an EMPI strategy for its planned merger with a 400-bed community hospital. Which characteristic of CAH operations most directly justifies EMPI investment? A) The 25-bed cap on inpatient beds B) The frequent transfer of patients to referral centers C) Cost-based Medicare reimbursement D) The 96-hour average length of stay rule **Answer: B** — CAHs by design stabilize and transfer; the frequent referral relationship makes identity reconciliation across organizational boundaries a clinical safety priority.

Systems Analysis

Exam Weight: 17% (range 15–19%)

Learning Objectives: - Apply structured analysis techniques — needs assessment, gap analysis, workflow analysis, root-cause analysis — to clinical and administrative IT problems. - Translate stakeholder needs into business and functional requirements using techniques appropriate to the audience. - Construct and interpret process models including swimlane diagrams, value stream maps, and BPMN diagrams. - Identify the artifacts produced during systems analysis and how each supports downstream design and selection. - Recognize common analysis pitfalls, including scope creep, requirements elicitation bias, and proxy-stakeholder substitution.

0.13 The Purpose of Systems Analysis

Systems analysis sits between problem identification and solution design. Its purpose is to convert a felt organizational pain — "documentation is taking too long," "denials are increasing," "lab results aren't reaching the inpatient team" — into a structured set of requirements that downstream design, selection, and implementation activities can satisfy. Skipping or shortcutting analysis is the single most common cause of failed health IT projects and a recurring CPHIMS exam theme. Candidates should be prepared for scenario items in which an organization "selected a system" before completing analysis and now suffers predictable consequences (cost overrun, user revolt, regulatory exposure).

The analyst's first task is to define the problem in the user's terms and then progressively translate those terms into language a vendor or developer can act on. A clinician saying "the system is slow" may mean any of: page load latency, login time, click count to complete an order, time to first useful response from a search, or simply that the workflow itself contains too many steps regardless of technology. Each diagnosis points to a different solution, and a competent analyst extracts the precise meaning through structured elicitation before recommending action.

0.14 Needs Assessment

A needs assessment establishes the scope of the problem and the current state of capability. Common techniques include stakeholder interviews, document review (policies, procedures, current workflows), direct observation (often called "Gemba walks" in lean practice), and quantitative analysis of existing data (audit logs, throughput reports, denial reports). The output is a needs statement that describes the gap between current state and a defined desired state.

A high-quality needs statement is specific, measurable, and time-bound. "Reduce inpatient discharge order to discharge time from a current average of 4.2 hours to a target of 2.0 hours by Q4" is actionable. "Improve discharge throughput" is not. CPHIMS exam items will test the candidate's ability to recognize the difference and select the needs statement that supports later requirements traceability.

0.15 Gap Analysis

Gap analysis compares the desired state to the current state along defined dimensions (people, process, technology, information, governance) and identifies the gaps that must be closed to reach the desired state. The "people" dimension assesses skills, staffing, and roles; "process" assesses workflows, policies, and procedures; "technology" assesses systems, infrastructure, and integrations; "information" assesses data availability, quality, and accessibility; "governance" assesses decision rights, oversight, and accountability structures.

A common analysis error is treating gap analysis as a technology-only exercise. If discharge delays are caused 60% by case-management staffing shortages and 30% by transportation arrangement bottlenecks, replacing the discharge planning module of the EHR will not move the metric. Exam items frequently present a scenario in which technology investment is proposed for a non-technology gap; the correct answer is to redirect the gap analysis or expand scope to address the dominant root cause.

0.16 Workflow Analysis

Workflow analysis documents the actual sequence of activities required to accomplish a process. Three notations dominate healthcare practice. Swimlane diagrams partition activities across actors (e.g., physician, nurse, lab tech, system) and time, making handoffs explicit. Value stream maps overlay cycle time and value-added time on each step, exposing non-value-added work that consumes capacity. Business Process Model and Notation (BPMN) is a more formal notation suitable for processes that will be modeled in workflow engines.

Workflow analysis must distinguish "work as imagined" (what policy says) from "work as done" (what staff actually do). Tracing the gap between the two is often the most valuable analyst contribution. A medication-reconciliation policy may specify that the admitting nurse complete reconciliation within four hours of admission using the EHR's home medication list; in practice the nurse may complete a paper form because the EHR's home medication list pre-populates with data the patient cannot confirm. The IT solution must address work as done, not work as imagined.

0.17 Requirements Elicitation and Documentation

Requirements come in three principal types. Business requirements describe what the organization wants to achieve (reduce discharge time, increase first-pass denial rate, comply with a new regulation). Functional requirements describe what the system must do to satisfy the business requirements (e.g., "the system shall display the discharge readiness scorecard on the inpatient unit dashboard, refreshing at intervals of no greater than 15 minutes"). Non-functional requirements describe how the system must behave (performance, availability, security, usability).

Elicitation techniques include interviews, focus groups, observation, document analysis, prototyping, and structured questionnaires. Each technique has a bias profile. Interviews surface what individuals are willing to say to a specific interviewer; focus groups surface consensus that may suppress dissenting views; observation surfaces actual behavior but cannot reveal motivation. The analyst should triangulate across techniques and document the source of every requirement so that later disputes can be resolved.

Requirements documentation should follow a consistent template. Each requirement gets a unique identifier, a statement, a source, an acceptance criterion, a priority (MoSCoW: Must, Should, Could, Won't), and a status. A traceability matrix maps each requirement to its source, its supporting design artifacts, its test cases, and the released code or configuration that implements it. Joint Commission and many state agencies require traceability for safety-critical systems.

0.18 Root-Cause Analysis

When a problem persists despite repeated intervention, root-cause analysis (RCA) is the appropriate technique. Common methods include the 5 Whys (iteratively asking why a condition exists), Ishikawa or fishbone diagrams (categorizing causes across people, methods, machines, materials, measurement, environment), and Fault Tree Analysis (deductively modeling the logic by which causes combine to produce an outcome).

In healthcare, sentinel events trigger mandatory RCA under Joint Commission requirements. The Joint Commission revised its sentinel event framework in 2024 to emphasize systems thinking and corrective action effectiveness over individual accountability. CPHIMS candidates should understand the RCA-to-action chain: an RCA without an action plan, an action plan without an owner and a date, and an action plan without effectiveness monitoring all fail Joint Commission expectations.

0.19 Common Analysis Pitfalls

Scope creep is the gradual expansion of project boundaries without corresponding adjustments to budget, schedule, or resources. The countermeasure is a formal change-control process and an explicit scope statement signed by sponsors. Requirements elicitation bias takes several forms: anchoring on the first solution suggested, vendor framing that constrains the requirements vocabulary to the vendor's product, and proxy-stakeholder substitution in which a manager speaks for the staff who actually perform the work. The proxy problem is endemic in healthcare IT; physicians frequently serve as proxies for nursing workflow analysis, and the resulting requirements miss the dominant clinical-operations drivers.

> **Exam Tip**
>
> When a question describes an IT project that failed despite "completing all requirements," look for an analysis-stage error: missing stakeholders, work-as-imagined requirements, or technology-only gap analysis.

> **Exam Tip**
>
> MoSCoW prioritization is the most commonly tested requirements-priority framework. Memorize: Must (non-negotiable for go-live), Should (high value but deferrable), Could (nice to have), Won't (this release).

> **Key Concept**
>
> Business requirements describe outcomes, functional requirements describe system behavior, and non-functional requirements describe operational qualities. The CPHIMS exam tests the candidate's ability to classify a given requirement into the correct type.

> **Key Concept**
>
> Workflow analysis must capture work as done, not work as imagined. Direct observation is the only technique that reliably reveals the difference.

> **Key Concept**
>
> Root cause analysis without an effectiveness check is incomplete. Joint Commission expects RCAs to document the action plan, owner, due date, and post-implementation effectiveness measure.

0.20 Chapter Review Questions

Q1. An IT director receives a complaint that "the EHR is slow." Which initial analysis activity will best clarify the actual problem? A) Increase server CPU allocation B) Conduct direct observation of clinicians using the EHR C) Engage the vendor for a performance audit D) Survey clinicians by email **Answer: B** — Direct observation reveals work as done, distinguishes infrastructure latency from workflow complexity, and allows the analyst to quantify click count, search-to-result latency, and other concrete measures.

Q2. Which requirements priority is reserved for items that are non-negotiable for the current release in the MoSCoW framework? A) Must B) Should C) Could D) Won't **Answer: A** — Must items are non-negotiable for the current release; failure to deliver any Must item is failure to deliver the release.

Q3. A health system completes gap analysis on discharge delays and identifies the dominant root cause as case-management staffing. Which response is most consistent with sound systems analysis practice? A) Recommend expanded EHR discharge module licensing anyway B) Refer the staffing finding to HR and document it as out of IT scope C) Expand the project charter and stakeholder set to include operations and finance D) Continue with technology-only requirements **Answer: C** — Gap analysis findings should drive project scope; a dominant non-technology cause requires expanding stakeholders rather than ignoring the finding or forcing a technology solution.

Q4. A sentinel event RCA identifies four causes and proposes four corrective actions. Which additional element does The Joint Commission require to consider the RCA complete? A) Disclosure to the patient's family B) An effectiveness measure for each corrective action C) Public posting of the RCA D) State health department notification **Answer: B** — The Joint Commission sentinel event framework requires that corrective actions include an effectiveness measure to confirm the action actually closed the gap; without it the RCA is incomplete.

Q5. Which requirement type does the following statement represent: "The system shall remain available 99.95% of the time during scheduled hours, measured monthly"? A) Business requirement B) Functional requirement C) Non-functional requirement D) Constraint **Answer: C** — Availability is a quality attribute of system operation and is therefore a non-functional requirement; functional requirements describe what the system does, not how reliably it does it.

Systems Design

Exam Weight: 12% (range 10–14%)

Learning Objectives: - Distinguish logical from physical design and identify the artifacts each produces. - Apply common architectural patterns (n-tier, microservices, integration-engine-mediated, API-led) to healthcare scenarios. - Design data models appropriate to clinical, financial, and analytic workloads, including dimensional models for warehousing. - Evaluate user-experience and usability principles applied to clinical software. - Specify integration designs using HL7 v2, FHIR (including SMART App Launch 2.1 and SMART Backend Services), IHE profiles, and modern API patterns. - Apply clinical decision support governance, including the HTI-1 DSI source attribute and Intervention Risk Management Practices requirements, to predictive AI/ML and evidence-based interventions, and recognize the FDA's PCCP framework for AI/ML SaMD.

0.21 Logical and Physical Design

Logical design specifies what the system will do without committing to specific technology choices. It produces data models, process models, user-interaction designs, and integration designs at a conceptual level. Physical design commits those conceptual models to specific platforms, databases, networks, and code organization. A well-run project completes logical design before physical design to avoid premature optimization and to preserve technology flexibility during procurement.

In healthcare, logical design must address clinical safety as a first-order concern. The design must specify how the system prevents and detects errors, including order conflicts, allergy violations, dosing errors, identity confusion, and result mis-routing. The IEC 62366 standard for medical-device usability and the FDA's premarket submission guidance on software functions both anchor logical-design expectations for clinical decision support, computerized order entry, and medication administration.

0.22 Architectural Patterns

Three architectural patterns dominate healthcare IT. Monolithic n-tier architectures, including the dominant inpatient EHR suites, organize the system into presentation, application, and data tiers, with all clinical and administrative functionality delivered from a single integrated stack. The benefit is workflow coherence; the cost is vendor lock-in and slow innovation cycles. Best-of-breed architectures combine specialized vendors for departmental needs (e.g., a separate cardiology IS, oncology IS, anesthesia IS) integrated through an integration engine. The benefit is functional depth; the cost is integration complexity and data-consistency challenges.

API-led and microservices architectures decompose functionality into services exposed through APIs, often using HL7 FHIR Release 4 as the canonical interchange format. The SMART on FHIR specification standardizes how third-party applications authenticate and authorize against a FHIR endpoint, enabling an app ecosystem analogous to mobile app stores. The benefit is innovation velocity and modular replacement; the cost is governance complexity around API contracts, performance, and security.

0.23 Data Modeling

Operational systems use normalized relational models optimized for transactional consistency. A typical hospital order has tables for the order, the patient, the ordering provider, the orderable item, the catalog entry, and audit trails. Normalization prevents anomalies during update but penalizes complex read queries — the model used for documenting an order is not the model used for analyzing 90 days of order patterns.

Analytic workloads use dimensional models, most commonly star schemas with fact and dimension tables. A fact table records measurable events (encounters, claims, lab results, medication administrations) with foreign keys to dimensions (patient, provider, location, time, payer). Conformed dimensions reused across fact tables enable cross-process analysis. The Kimball methodology dominates healthcare analytic modeling; the Inmon hub-and-spoke approach appears in larger integrated delivery networks with mature enterprise data warehouses.

OMOP (Observational Medical Outcomes Partnership) Common Data Model has become the de facto standard for cross-institution research and increasingly for operational analytics. OMOP standardizes vocabularies (using SNOMED CT, RxNorm, LOINC) and physical structure across implementations, enabling research networks like OHDSI to run identical analytic protocols across hundreds of sites. CPHIMS candidates should know that OMOP is a research-anchored model and is not optimized for operational reporting; many organizations maintain both an operational warehouse and an OMOP mart.

0.24 Master Data and Identity

Master data management (MDM) in healthcare includes the patient master (handled by the EMPI), the provider master (handled by the EPDM or provider data management system), the location master, the catalog master (orderables, charge codes, supply items), and the payer master. Each master must define a survival rule for conflicting source values, an attribute-level provenance, and a publication mechanism to downstream consumers.

Patient identity is the most operationally sensitive master domain. EMPI matching uses deterministic rules for exact matches on a defined set of attributes (e.g., name + DOB + SSN), probabilistic algorithms that compute a match score across many attributes, and referential matching against external identity sources. A well-tuned EMPI achieves 99%+ true positive rate at less than 0.01% false positive rate, but tuning is iterative and ongoing.

EMPI threshold design has two principal forms candidates should recognize. A single-threshold design treats every candidate match above the threshold as an automatic link and every candidate match below as a reject (no manual queue). A two-threshold design defines an upper threshold (auto-link), a lower threshold (auto-reject), and a manual-review band in between. Lowering thresholds in a single-threshold design increases auto-links and decreases manual review only because there is no manual band; lowering the upper threshold in a two-threshold design typically increases auto-links and may also increase, decrease, or leave unchanged the manual band depending on how the two thresholds move relative to one another. CPHIMS items may test this distinction; candidates should read scenario stems carefully for explicit threshold-design assumptions.

0.25 User Experience and Usability

Clinical software usability is a measurable patient-safety variable. The ISO 9241-11 definition — effectiveness, efficiency, and satisfaction — applies, but in clinical settings safety is the dominant criterion. Common usability defects include alert fatigue (excessive low-specificity alerts causing clinicians to ignore all alerts including high-specificity safety alerts), modal interruption fatigue (similar pattern with modal pop-ups), excessive click count for routine tasks, and information density that exceeds working-memory capacity.

The Office of the National Coordinator's Safety Assurance Factors for EHR Resilience (SAFER) Guides specify usability and safety practices across nine domains. The Computerized Physician Order Entry with Decision Support guide is the most frequently cited and lists specific recommended practices that exam items may reference. The 2024 update to SAFER added guidance on clinical decision support governance and the use of probabilistic AI in clinical workflows.

0.26 Clinical Decision Support Governance for Predictive Models

Clinical decision support (CDS) governance is no longer optional under federal regulation for organizations using certified Health IT. The HTI-1 Final Rule's Decision Support Intervention (DSI) certification criterion at 45 CFR 170.315(b)(11) divides CDS into two classes — evidence-based and predictive — and applies progressively stronger source attribute and risk management obligations to predictive interventions.

For evidence-based DSI (a clinical rule grounded in published evidence or organizational policy), the source attribute disclosures cover the rule's purpose, source(s), reference(s), and known limitations. For predictive DSI (a rule whose output depends on a predictive model, including AI/ML models), the source attribute disclosures cover an expanded list: the intervention's purpose and intended use; the underlying data used to develop the model; the input variables used at run time; the output produced and how it is to be used; the training and validation populations including demographic representation; performance metrics on validation data; fairness measures across subpopulations; security and integrity protections; and ongoing post-deployment monitoring practices.

The Intervention Risk Management Practice (IRMP) is the developer-side governance instrument. An IRMP documents the risk analysis the developer performs before deploying the DSI, the risk mitigation steps the developer takes, and the developer's ongoing monitoring and retirement criteria. The developer must publish a summary of its IRMP. Healthcare organizations deploying DSI within certified products must establish a corresponding deployment-side governance practice that uses the developer's source attribute disclosures, monitors local performance, and retires or adjusts interventions whose performance degrades.

Predictive DSI deployment in healthcare is also affected by the FDA's framework for AI/ML-enabled Software as a Medical Device (SaMD). The FDA finalized its Predetermined Change Control Plan (PCCP) guidance in December 2024. A PCCP is a documented plan submitted as part of a premarket submission that describes specific, anticipated modifications a manufacturer may make to an AI/ML-enabled device after authorization — including changes to the model, the training data set, and performance characteristics — without a new premarket submission for each modification. PCCP guidance establishes the framework for "locked" versus "adaptive" AI/ML SaMD and the manufacturer's obligations for change protocols, change validation, and post-market monitoring. CPHIMS candidates should recognize PCCP as the FDA's response to the rapid iteration cycle of AI/ML and should distinguish FDA-regulated AI/ML SaMD from non-device CDS that falls under HTI-1 alone.

0.27 Integration Design

Integration design specifies how systems exchange data. Three patterns dominate. Point-to-point integration directly connects pairs of systems and is appropriate only for the smallest environments because the connection count grows as n(n-1)/2. Integration-engine-mediated architectures route HL7 v2 messages through a hub (Iguana, Rhapsody, Cloverleaf, Mirth/NextGen Connect) that handles routing, transformation, and queueing. API-led integration exposes functionality through FHIR or proprietary REST APIs and emphasizes synchronous request-response patterns rather than asynchronous message flows.

For FHIR-based integration, two SMART specifications matter at the exam level. SMART App Launch 2.1.0 (May 2024) is the current widely-deployed version of the user-facing app-launch profile; it standardizes how third-party clinical apps obtain OAuth 2.0 authorization to read or write FHIR resources on behalf of a clinician or patient user. SMART Backend Services standardizes system-to-system FHIR exchange with no human user — typically used for CMS Bulk Data exports, payer-provider Da Vinci flows, and population-level analytics. Backend Services uses asymmetric key cryptography (JWS-signed client assertions) for client authentication rather than the OAuth 2.0 redirect flows used by App Launch.

IHE (Integrating the Healthcare Enterprise) profiles bundle standards into reusable use-case implementations. PIX/PDQ (Patient Identifier Cross-Reference / Patient Demographics Query) standardizes patient identity exchange. XDS (Cross-Enterprise Document Sharing) standardizes document exchange. ATNA (Audit Trail and Node Authentication) standardizes audit logging across systems. The IHE Connectathon and HIMSS Interoperability Showcase validate vendor implementations annually.

> **Exam Tip**
>
> A best-of-breed architecture is not inherently superior to a monolithic architecture. Exam items test whether candidates can match architectural pattern to organizational context (size, integration capability, change tolerance, vendor strategy).

> **Exam Tip**
>
> When an item asks about EMPI tuning, distinguish single-threshold from two-threshold designs and remember that increasing automatic linking always increases the false-positive risk regardless of design.

> **Exam Tip**
>
> A FHIR-flavored item that mentions "system-to-system" or "no user present" implicates SMART Backend Services rather than SMART App Launch. App Launch implicates an OAuth 2.0 redirect flow with a human user.

> **Key Concept**
>
> Logical design produces conceptual artifacts independent of specific technology; physical design commits those artifacts to chosen platforms. Conflating the two is the most common cause of premature lock-in.

> **Key Concept**
>
> SMART on FHIR is the dominant standard for third-party clinical app authentication and authorization against an FHIR endpoint. SMART App Launch 2.1 (user-facing) and SMART Backend Services (system-to-system) are both current and exam-relevant.

> **Key Concept**
>
> Star-schema dimensional modeling, popularized by the Kimball methodology, remains the most common analytic data model in healthcare. OMOP is the de facto research standard.

> **Key Concept**
>
> Predictive DSI deployment requires source attribute review (per HTI-1), local governance, and ongoing performance monitoring. FDA-regulated AI/ML SaMD additionally requires conformance to the PCCP framework if the manufacturer wants to modify the model post-authorization.

0.28 Chapter Review Questions

Q1. Which architectural pattern minimizes integration complexity at the cost of slow innovation cycles and vendor lock-in? A) Microservices B) Monolithic n-tier C) API-led D) Best-of-breed **Answer: B** — Monolithic n-tier architectures (including major inpatient EHR suites) deliver workflow coherence with low integration overhead but slow innovation cycles and create vendor lock-in.

Q2. A health system implements SMART on FHIR to support a clinical decision support app marketplace that launches inside the clinician's EHR session. Which SMART profile and authentication flow apply? A) SMART App Launch 2.1 with OAuth 2.0 authorization code flow B) SMART Backend Services with JWS client assertion C) HTTP Basic Authentication D) HTTP Digest Authentication **Answer: A** — SMART App Launch 2.1 with OAuth 2.0 authorization code flow standardizes user-facing third-party app launch from within a clinician (or patient) session; Backend Services is the system-to-system equivalent and uses JWS-signed client assertions.

Q3. A research network plans to run identical analytic protocols across 80 hospital sites. Which data model is most appropriate as the common target? A) Kimball star schema operational warehouse B) OMOP Common Data Model C) HL7 v2 inbound message archive D) Hospital-specific normalized clinical model **Answer: B** — OMOP standardizes both physical structure and clinical vocabulary across implementations, enabling research networks to run identical analyses across institutions.

Q4. Which usability defect most directly contributes to clinicians ignoring high-specificity safety alerts in the EHR? A) Excessive click count B) Information density C) Alert fatigue from low-specificity alerts D) Modal interruption **Answer: C** — Alert fatigue is the documented and SAFER-Guide-recognized phenomenon in which a high volume of low-specificity alerts trains clinicians to dismiss alerts reflexively, eroding the value of high-specificity safety alerts.

Q5. Which IHE profile standardizes patient identifier cross-reference across enterprises? A) XDS B) ATNA C) PIX D) XCA **Answer: C** — PIX (Patient Identifier Cross-Reference) standardizes the mapping of patient identifiers across enterprises; PDQ (Patient Demographics Query) is its demographic-query counterpart.

Systems Selection, Implementation, Support, and Maintenance

Exam Weight: 24% (range 21–27%)

Learning Objectives: - Conduct a structured vendor selection from RFI through contract execution. - Plan and govern an implementation project using waterfall, agile, and hybrid methodologies. - Define and manage support tiers, SLAs, and operational ownership for a clinical system. - Manage release, upgrade, and patch processes against a clinical risk framework. - Apply standard project management concepts (scope, schedule, budget, risk, communication, procurement) in the healthcare context.

0.29 Vendor Selection

Vendor selection begins after analysis has produced a validated requirements set and ends with a signed contract. The standard sequence is market scan, request for information (RFI), request for proposal (RFP) or request for quote (RFQ), vendor demonstrations, reference checks, due diligence, and contract negotiation. Each step is gated by an explicit decision and documented criteria.

Market scan identifies the vendors who could plausibly satisfy the requirements. KLAS Research, Black Book, and Gartner reports inform the scan but should not substitute for primary research; rankings reflect a specific evaluation methodology that may not match the organization's priorities. The RFI elicits high-level vendor capability and is appropriate for narrowing a long list. The RFP is a binding solicitation tied to a defined scope, evaluation criteria, and timeline. The RFP must publish the scoring rubric in advance so vendors can target their responses and so the evaluation team can defend its decision.

Vendor demonstrations must be scripted. An unstructured demo lets the vendor showcase strengths and bury weaknesses. A scripted demo presents standardized clinical scenarios the vendor must demonstrate live, ideally using the prospect's own data after a sanitization process. Reference checks should target customers similar to the prospect in size, complexity, and time-since-implementation. References within the first six months of go-live are unreliable; references at 18 months reveal sustained performance and vendor responsiveness.

Due diligence assesses vendor financial stability, security posture (SOC 2 Type II reports, HITRUST CSF certification, penetration test summaries), regulatory compliance (ONC Certified Health IT for EHR functions, current HTI-1 conformance for products that include DSI), and contractual flexibility. The contract should address data ownership and return at termination, performance SLAs with credits, change-control procedures, source code escrow for critical systems, and breach notification timelines that satisfy HIPAA and state law.

0.30 Implementation Methodologies

Waterfall implementations sequence analysis, design, build, test, and deploy as distinct phases with formal gate reviews. Waterfall remains appropriate for tightly regulated workflows where each phase must be fully validated before the next begins, including FDA-regulated medical-device software (under IEC 62304) and many clinical-trial systems. The risk is that defects discovered late are expensive to correct.

Agile implementations deliver functionality in short iterations (typically two-to-four-week sprints) that produce working software at the end of each iteration. The framework most common in healthcare IT is Scrum, with roles for Product Owner, Scrum Master, and Development Team. Agile is appropriate for greenfield projects where requirements are uncertain and stakeholder feedback shapes priorities. The risk in healthcare is that some workflow integrations cannot be partially deployed; a clinical documentation system that supports only half of a unit's workflow may be worse than the status quo.

Hybrid methodologies, including SAFe (Scaled Agile Framework), apply waterfall governance to scope, schedule, and budget while using agile execution within work streams. Many enterprise EHR projects use a hybrid: waterfall governance for the overall program with agile sprints inside specific application teams (e.g., the ED implementation team or the ambulatory specialty configuration team).

Big-bang versus phased deployment is a separate question from methodology. Big-bang implementations cut over all sites or modules at a single point in time, requiring substantial command-center support but eliminating dual-state operations. Phased deployment reduces concurrent risk but creates dual-system operations that strain integrations and reporting.

0.31 Project Management Discipline

The Project Management Institute's PMBOK framework identifies ten knowledge areas: integration, scope, schedule, cost, quality, resource, communications, risk, procurement, and stakeholder. CPHIMS exam items frequently test scope, schedule, cost, risk, and stakeholder management.

Scope management requires a documented scope statement, a work breakdown structure (WBS), and a change-control procedure. WBS decomposes the project into deliverables and work packages, with no work package exceeding the 80-hour 8/80 rule for granularity. Change control logs each scope-change request, assesses impact on schedule and cost, and routes approval to the appropriate authority.

Schedule management uses critical-path or critical-chain methods to identify the longest sequence of dependent tasks. Schedule compression techniques include fast-tracking (parallelizing tasks formerly sequenced) and crashing (adding resources to compress duration). Both have risks: fast-tracking increases rework risk; crashing produces diminishing returns and may not reduce duration at all on already resource-loaded tasks.

Cost management requires a documented budget at WBS-work-package level, an earned value tracking method, and variance thresholds that trigger corrective action. Earned value uses Planned Value (PV), Earned Value (EV), and Actual Cost (AC) to compute Schedule Variance (EV – PV), Cost Variance (EV – AC), Schedule Performance Index (EV / PV), and Cost Performance Index (EV / AC). An SPI of 0.85 means the project has delivered 85% of the value planned to date; a CPI of 0.85 means the project spent 100 dollars to deliver 85 dollars of value.

Risk management identifies risks proactively, assesses probability and impact, and assigns owners and responses. The four standard risk responses are Avoid, Transfer, Mitigate, and Accept (ATMA). For implementations, the highest-impact risk categories are clinical safety, regulatory non-compliance, data integrity at conversion, and stakeholder resistance.

0.32 Support Operations

Once a system goes live, support operations take over from the project team. Support is typically tiered. Tier 1 handles password resets, basic user questions, and access requests. Tier 2 handles application configuration, complex workflow questions, and minor break-fix. Tier 3 handles vendor escalation, deep technical investigation, and infrastructure issues. The boundaries between tiers must be documented in a support model and reinforced through training; ill-defined boundaries cause Tier 1 to escalate prematurely or Tier 3 to absorb work below its skill level.

Service level agreements should specify response time (time to acknowledge), restoration time (time to restore service), and resolution time (time to permanent fix) for each severity level. Severity 1 incidents — system down for clinical operations — typically require response within 15 minutes and restoration within four hours; the exact targets vary by contract and by organizational risk tolerance.

ITIL v4 is the dominant service management framework in healthcare IT. CPHIMS candidates should know the incident management, problem management, change management, and release management processes. Problem management is the practice of identifying the root cause of recurring incidents and is distinct from incident management, which focuses on service restoration.

0.33 Maintenance, Upgrades, and Patches

EHR vendors release updates on schedules ranging from quarterly to multiple-times-yearly. Major releases may include workflow changes that require physician and nursing retraining; minor releases and patches typically focus on bug fixes and security updates. The organization must maintain a release management process that classifies each update by clinical risk, schedules deployment in a non-production environment for validation, validates against a defined test plan, and obtains clinical and operational sign-off before production deployment.

Patch management for security vulnerabilities follows a different cadence. Critical vulnerabilities (CVSS 9.0 and above) require emergency change procedures and may bypass standard release windows. Organizations should maintain a documented patch SLA — for example, critical patches within 14 days, high within 30, medium within 60 — and report compliance to leadership.

0.34 Downtime Planning and Testing

Downtime planning is a Joint Commission Information Management chapter expectation, and CMS Conditions of Participation include emergency preparedness requirements that apply to clinical IT. Operationally, every hospital must have documented downtime procedures covering planned outages (releases, maintenance windows) and unplanned outages (system failure, network failure, ransomware), with clinical paper forms and printed reference data available for the duration. The CMS Emergency Preparedness Rule requires healthcare organizations to conduct at least annual exercises that test the emergency operations plan, and many organizations supplement the annual exercise with periodic tabletop exercises and unit-level drills throughout the year. The Joint Commission Emergency Management (EM) and Information Management (IM) standards do not specify a quarterly cadence; the operational baseline is an annual full exercise with periodic tabletops and unit-level drills, and organizations vary their additional cadence based on local risk assessment. CPHIMS candidates should not assume quarterly full-failover testing is a Joint Commission requirement.

0.35 Decommissioning

End-of-life decommissioning is the most overlooked phase of system lifecycle. Decommissioning must address data retention, data migration to a successor or archive system, contractual cleanup, license termination, infrastructure return or destruction, and user communication. HIPAA, state retention laws, and ongoing litigation holds may require data retention for many years past system retirement. A decommissioning plan should identify each obligation, the retention period, and the storage strategy (often a dedicated legal/medical archive system).

> **Exam Tip**
>
> The exam frequently tests the distinction between incident management (restore service) and problem management (find and fix root cause). Memorize: an incident is a service disruption, a problem is the underlying cause, and a known error is a problem with a documented workaround.

> **Exam Tip**
>
> Earned Value Management acronyms (PV, EV, AC, SV, CV, SPI, CPI) are high-frequency exam topics. An SPI or CPI below 1.0 indicates performance behind plan.

> **Key Concept**
>
> Vendor demos must be scripted and reference checks must target peers at 18+ months post-go-live. Unstructured demos and early-go-live references are the two highest-yield selection errors.

> **Key Concept**
>
> Waterfall, agile, and hybrid methodologies each have a context where they excel. CPHIMS items test the candidate's ability to match methodology to context, not to argue universally for one approach.

> **Key Concept**
>
> Decommissioning is part of lifecycle, not an afterthought. HIPAA data retention obligations may extend years past system retirement.

0.36 Chapter Review Questions

Q1. A health system is selecting an oncology information system. Reference checks should target organizations that match the prospect on which dimension? A) Geographic region B) Time since go-live (at least 18 months) C) Number of vendor employees D) Cloud versus on-premises deployment **Answer: B** — References within the first six months of go-live are unreliable because the implementation team is still on site; 18-month references reveal sustained performance and vendor responsiveness.

Q2. A project reports an SPI of 0.92 and a CPI of 1.05 at the midpoint review. What is the correct interpretation? A) The project is ahead of schedule and over budget B) The project is behind schedule and under budget C) The project is on schedule and under budget D) The project is behind schedule and over budget **Answer: B** — SPI below 1.0 indicates schedule delay; CPI above 1.0 indicates cost performance better than plan.

Q3. Which ITIL process is responsible for identifying and addressing the root cause of recurring incidents? A) Incident Management B) Change Management C) Problem Management D) Service Request Management **Answer: C** — Problem Management addresses root cause; Incident Management focuses on service restoration.

Q4. A critical vendor security patch addresses a CVSS 9.6 vulnerability in the EHR's authentication service. Which release management approach is most appropriate? A) Wait for the next scheduled quarterly release B) Apply through emergency change procedures with abbreviated validation C) Defer until the vendor publishes a non-security release D) Skip the patch and apply compensating controls **Answer: B** — Critical CVSS vulnerabilities (9.0+) require emergency change procedures; standard release windows are bypassed but validation is performed at an abbreviated but defined level.

Q5. A clinical system is being decommissioned after 12 years. Which obligation most directly drives data retention requirements? A) Vendor contractual minimum B) HIPAA and state record retention laws C) Industry best practice D) IT department storage policy **Answer: B** — HIPAA Privacy Rule requirements and applicable state record retention laws set the binding minimum for clinical data retention after system retirement.

Systems Privacy and Security

Exam Weight: 12% (range 10–14%)

Learning Objectives: - Apply the HIPAA Privacy Rule, Security Rule, Breach Notification Rule, and the December 2024 Security Rule NPRM to operational scenarios. - Distinguish administrative, physical, and technical safeguards and provide examples of each. - Apply identity and access management principles, including authentication, authorization, role-based and attribute-based access control, and provisioning lifecycle, with appropriate use of NIST SP 800-63B AAL terminology. - Conduct or interpret risk analysis under 45 CFR 164.308(a)(1)(ii)(A). - Manage incident response and breach notification under the 60-day notice clock.

0.37 The HIPAA Regulatory Framework

The HIPAA Privacy Rule (45 CFR Part 160 and Part 164 Subparts A and E) governs the use and disclosure of Protected Health Information (PHI). PHI is individually identifiable health information held or transmitted by a covered entity (health plan, healthcare clearinghouse, or healthcare provider that conducts certain electronic transactions) or its business associate. The Privacy Rule defines permitted uses and disclosures (for treatment, payment, healthcare operations, and several specified public-interest purposes), required disclosures (to the individual on request and to the Secretary of HHS for compliance investigations), and authorization-required disclosures (all others).

The Security Rule (45 CFR Part 160 and Part 164 Subparts A and C) governs the confidentiality, integrity, and availability of electronic PHI (ePHI). The rule organizes safeguards into administrative (45 CFR 164.308), physical (164.310), and technical (164.312) categories, each with required and addressable implementation specifications. "Addressable" does not mean optional; a covered entity must implement the specification, document a reasonable alternative that achieves the same objective, or document why neither is reasonable for its environment.

In December 2024, OCR published a Notice of Proposed Rulemaking (NPRM) proposing the first major Security Rule update since 2013. The NPRM proposes to remove the addressable/required distinction (all specifications become required), to require multi-factor authentication for access to ePHI, to require encryption of ePHI at rest and in transit with specified algorithm strength, to require annual penetration testing and vulnerability scanning at defined intervals, and to expand contingency planning requirements. **As of the most recent public record this NPRM has not been finalized; the comment period closed in March 2025 and a final rule has not yet been published. Candidates should monitor the HHS Office for Civil Rights (OCR) and the Federal Register for finalization and should not assume any portion of the NPRM is in force.** Candidates who memorize a non-existent final rule risk missing exam items.

The Breach Notification Rule (45 CFR 164.400–414) requires notification to affected individuals within 60 days of discovery of a breach involving unsecured PHI. A breach involving more than 500 residents of a state or jurisdiction requires immediate notification to OCR and to prominent media. Breaches affecting fewer than 500 individuals are reported to OCR annually no later than 60 days after the end of the calendar year.

HITECH established a four-tier civil money penalty structure that distinguishes the violator's culpability: Tier 1 (lack of knowledge), Tier 2 (reasonable cause and not willful neglect), Tier 3 (willful neglect, corrected within 30 days), and Tier 4 (willful neglect, not corrected). Each tier has its own per-violation minimum, per-violation maximum, and per-calendar-year cap for repeat violations of the same provision. HHS adjusts the amounts annually for inflation; the most recent formal inflation adjustment was published in the Federal Register in November 2024. As of that adjustment, the Tier 4 per-violation maximum and the per year cap for repeat Tier 4 violations are in the low millions of dollars, while Tier 1 maximums are substantially lower. Candidates should not memorize a single dollar figure; instead memorize the four-tier structure, recognize that HHS updates the figures annually, and look up the current Federal Register figures during their final pre-exam review.

0.38 Risk Analysis

The Security Rule requires covered entities to conduct an accurate and thorough assessment of potential risks and vulnerabilities to ePHI (45 CFR 164.308(a)(1)(ii)(A)) and to implement security measures sufficient to reduce risks to a reasonable and appropriate level. Risk analysis is not a one-time activity; it must be repeated when the environment changes materially (new system deployment, organizational restructure, identified vulnerability) and at least annually as a best practice.

NIST SP 800-66 Revision 2 (published 2024) provides the most current implementation guidance for HIPAA Security Rule risk analysis. The standard risk analysis process identifies assets, identifies threats and vulnerabilities, assesses current security controls, determines likelihood and impact, calculates risk, identifies risk responses, and documents the analysis. The output is a risk register that tracks each identified risk, its current state, the planned response, and the residual risk. The NIST Cybersecurity Framework 2.0 (Feb 2024) provides complementary structure for security program maturity: organizations commonly map their HIPAA Security Rule controls to CSF Categories and Subcategories using the NIST-published HIPAA-to-CSF crosswalk.

0.39 Identity and Access Management

Authentication establishes who a user is. The 2024 Security Rule NPRM and OCR enforcement actions through 2025 have effectively established multi-factor authentication (MFA) as the operational baseline for ePHI access; single-factor passwords for clinical access are an OCR enforcement risk.

NIST SP 800-63B identifies three Authenticator Assurance Levels (AAL1, AAL2, AAL3). AAL1 permits single-factor authentication. AAL2 requires two factors and is the practical baseline for clinical systems; AAL2 authenticators may include phishing-vulnerable factors such as SMS one-time-passcodes, push notifications, or memorized secrets paired with a separate factor. AAL3 requires the use of hardware-based authenticators and explicitly requires phishing-resistant verifier impersonation resistance — properties typically achieved by FIDO2/WebAuthn security keys, PIV cards, or equivalent hardware-bound credentials. NIST reserves the term "phishing-resistant" for AAL3-class authenticators; conflating AAL2 with "phishing-resistant" is a common error.

For 2026-current healthcare practice: AAL2 with strong factors is the practical baseline; phishing-resistant authenticators (AAL3-class) are recommended for high-risk roles, privileged administrator access, and any role with broad PHI access, consistent with recent OCR enforcement guidance and the direction signaled by the December 2024 Security Rule NPRM. CPHIMS candidates should be able to distinguish AAL2 from AAL3 and recognize the language "phishing-resistant" as an AAL3-class property.

Authorization establishes what an authenticated user may do. Role-based access control (RBAC) assigns permissions to roles and roles to users. Attribute-based access control (ABAC) computes access decisions from user attributes, resource attributes, and environmental attributes (time, location, device posture). Most large EHRs use RBAC for routine access with ABAC overlays for context-sensitive scenarios (break-glass, VIP access, sensitive specialty).

Provisioning lifecycle management — joiner, mover, leaver (JML) — is a frequent OCR audit finding when poorly executed. Stale accounts of terminated employees and over-privileged accounts of moved employees are leading causes of insider breach. Automated provisioning tied to HR system events is the operational standard for organizations above ~500 staff; smaller organizations may rely on documented manual processes.

0.40 Encryption and Data Protection

Encryption of ePHI at rest and in transit is "addressable" under the current Security Rule and would become explicitly required if the December 2024 NPRM is finalized as proposed. As of 2026 the addressable status remains in force; nevertheless, OCR enforcement practice has effectively treated unencrypted ePHI as a per-se compliance gap. AES-256 for symmetric encryption at rest and TLS 1.2 or 1.3 for transit are the operational standards. Key management — generation, storage, rotation, retirement — must be addressed in the security program; encryption with poorly managed keys provides limited protection.

De-identification removes a defined set of identifiers from PHI to convert it to non-PHI for permitted uses such as research and quality reporting. The Privacy Rule provides two methods. The Safe Harbor method removes 18 specified identifier types (45 CFR 164.514(b)(2)). The Expert Determination method certifies through statistical analysis that the residual re-identification risk is very small. The Safe Harbor method is administratively simpler; the Expert Determination method preserves more analytic utility for advanced uses.

A Limited Data Set (LDS) removes a smaller set of identifiers than Safe Harbor and may include dates and limited geography. An LDS is still PHI but may be disclosed for research, public health, or healthcare operations under a Data Use Agreement (DUA).

0.41 Audit Logging and Monitoring

The Security Rule requires audit controls (164.312(b)) to record and examine activity in information systems containing ePHI. Logs should capture authentication events, authorization decisions, access to specific records, and administrative actions. Log review is the operational counterpart to log generation; logs that no one reviews provide compliance documentation but no real detection capability. The IHE ATNA profile standardizes audit event format and transport and underpins many enterprise audit aggregation systems.

Specific monitoring scenarios are recurring OCR enforcement themes: VIP record access by staff without a treatment relationship, employee access to records of family or neighbors, and disproportionate record access patterns (a clinician opening 200 records per shift versus a peer-average of 30). User behavior analytics (UBA) tools detect anomalous patterns automatically; for smaller organizations, sampled targeted audits remain the operational baseline. When a user is properly authenticated and the role's permission set allows the access, audit and analytics — not authentication or authorization — are the detective controls that flag the violation.

0.42 Incident Response and Breach Notification

Incident response begins with detection. Once an incident is suspected, the organization must contain the incident, investigate, determine whether a breach of unsecured PHI occurred, and execute notifications within the 60-day clock if a breach is confirmed. The Breach Risk Assessment under the Omnibus Rule requires consideration of four factors: the nature and extent of the PHI involved, the unauthorized person who used or received the PHI, whether the PHI was actually acquired or viewed, and the extent to which the risk has been mitigated.

A breach involving 500 or more residents of a state or jurisdiction triggers: notification to affected individuals within 60 days, notification to OCR within 60 days, and notification to prominent media in the affected geography within 60 days. Penalties for HIPAA violations follow the four-tier civil money penalty structure described above, with HHS adjusting per-tier minimums, maximums, and per-year caps annually for inflation.

Exam Tip

"Addressable" in the HIPAA Security Rule never means optional. A covered entity must implement the specification, implement a documented alternative that achieves the objective, or document why neither is reasonable.

Exam Tip

The breach notification clock is 60 days from discovery, not from occurrence. CPHIMS items test the candidate's understanding of when the clock starts.

Exam Tip

NIST reserves "phishing-resistant" language for AAL3 authenticators. AAL2 may include phishing-vulnerable factors (SMS OTP, push notifications). If a stem describes "phishing-resistant authenticators," think AAL3.

Key Concept

The Security Rule's three safeguard categories — administrative, physical, technical — apply to every CPHIMS analysis of a security control gap. Memorize representative examples in each category.

Key Concept

Risk analysis is recurring, not one-time. Material environmental change triggers reanalysis regardless of calendar timing.

Key Concept

Authentication, authorization, and auditing form the IAM triad. CPHIMS items frequently test the candidate's ability to identify which is failing in a scenario (an unauthorized user successfully accessing a record indicates an authorization gap that audit and analytics then detect, not an authentication failure, when the user authenticated under a valid identity).

Key Concept

HIPAA penalties follow a four-tier structure inflation-adjusted annually by HHS. Memorize the four tiers and verify current figures in the Federal Register near exam time.

0.43 Chapter Review Questions

Q1. A covered entity discovers on March 1 that an unauthorized employee accessed 800 patient records on January 15. By what date must individual notifications be sent under the Breach Notification Rule? A) March 17 B) April 30 C) March 31 D) January 60 days after the incident occurred **Answer: B** — The 60-day notification clock starts at discovery (March 1), making the latest notification date April 30; the clock does not start at the date of the underlying access event.

Q2. Which HIPAA Security Rule safeguard category does workforce training fall under? A) Administrative B) Physical C) Technical D) Procedural **Answer: A** — Workforce security training is an administrative safeguard required under 45 CFR 164.308(a)(5); the Security Rule's three safeguard categories are administrative, physical, and technical.

Q3. A clinician with valid credentials accesses the record of a celebrity admitted to the hospital without a treatment relationship. Which IAM function did the access most directly violate? A) Authentication B) Authorization C) Auditing D) Provisioning **Answer: B** — The clinician authenticated under a valid identity but was not authorized to access this specific record; the failure is one of authorization (and downstream audit/analytics detection), not authentication.

Q4. Under the HIPAA Privacy Rule Safe Harbor de-identification method, how many specified identifier types must be removed? A) 8 B) 12 C) 18 D) 24 **Answer: C** — Safe Harbor de-identification at 45 CFR 164.514(b)(2) requires removal of 18 specified identifier types; the Expert Determination method is the alternative for organizations preserving analytic utility.

Q5. Which NIST publication provides the most current implementation guidance for HIPAA Security Rule risk analysis? A) NIST SP 800-53 Revision 5 B) NIST SP 800-66 Revision 2 C) NIST SP 800-171 Revision 3 D) NIST Cybersecurity Framework 2.0 **Answer: B** — NIST SP 800-66 Revision 2, published in February 2024, is the authoritative HIPAA Security Rule implementation guide; the Cybersecurity Framework 2.0 and 800-53 are complementary but not HIPAA-specific.

Administration, Leadership, and Management

Exam Weight: 12% (range 10–14%)

Learning Objectives: - Apply IT governance principles, including portfolio management, project prioritization, and IT steering committee structures. - Develop and manage IT operating and capital budgets in a healthcare context, including TCO and ROI analysis. - Lead and develop IT staff including organizational design, performance management, and succession planning. - Communicate effectively with executive, clinical, operational, and external stakeholders. - Apply change management frameworks (ADKAR, Kotter, Prosci) to clinical IT initiatives.

0.44 IT Governance

IT governance is the structure of decision rights and accountability for IT investment and operation. In healthcare, IT governance must reconcile clinical, operational, financial, and regulatory priorities under finite resource constraints. The standard structure includes an IT steering committee or technology committee chaired by a senior executive (CIO, COO, or CEO) and including clinical, operational, and financial leaders. The committee approves the IT portfolio, sets investment priorities, reviews major project status, and adjudicates resource conflicts.

Portfolio management evaluates the set of all proposed and active IT initiatives against organizational priorities and resource availability. Portfolio scoring rubrics typically include strategic alignment, financial return, clinical safety impact, regulatory compliance, risk, and feasibility. A well-run portfolio rejects more proposals than it approves; rejection discipline is a measurable governance maturity indicator.

COBIT 2019 is the dominant IT governance framework and is recognized by Joint Commission surveyors and CMS auditors as evidence of mature IT management. COBIT identifies governance objectives (EDM domain) distinct from management objectives (APO, BAI, DSS, MEA domains). Healthcare-specific guidance, including the HIMSS Davies Award case studies, complements general IT governance with clinical-context examples.

0.45 Financial Management

Healthcare IT operates within two distinct financial frames: operating expense (OpEx) and capital expense (CapEx). Cloud subscriptions, support contracts, and staff salaries are OpEx; on-premises infrastructure and major software licenses have historically been CapEx, though the cloud shift has moved much of the spend to OpEx and required CFO partnership to maintain board comfort with growing run-rate.

Total Cost of Ownership (TCO) accounts for direct acquisition cost plus implementation cost, training, ongoing licensing, support, infrastructure, integration, and end-of-life decommissioning over the system's economic life. CPHIMS candidates should know that vendor list price typically represents 15–25% of seven-year TCO; analysis based on list price alone is a frequent decision-making error.

Return on Investment (ROI) measures financial return against investment. The basic formula is (Benefit – Cost) / Cost × 100%. Healthcare ROI calculations should distinguish hard savings (measurable expense reductions or revenue gains), soft savings (productivity improvements without head-count change), and avoidance (revenue or cost not incurred relative to a counterfactual baseline). Hard savings are credible to finance; soft savings and avoidance require defensible measurement methodology to be accepted.

The healthcare IT budget should track to a chargeback or showback model that attributes IT cost to consuming departments. Chargeback creates direct accountability but adds administrative overhead and may drive shadow IT; showback informs without billing. Most academic medical centers operate showback at the service-line level.

0.46 Leadership and Workforce Management

Healthcare IT organizations are typically structured along a combination of functional (application, infrastructure, security, project management, analytics) and customer (ambulatory, inpatient, ancillary) axes. The matrix structure is common but adds management complexity; clarity of decision rights between functional and customer leaders prevents the matrix from becoming a finger-pointing structure.

Workforce planning must address recruitment, retention, development, and succession. Healthcare IT competes for talent with banking, e-commerce, and pure technology employers; compensation parity at the senior individual contributor level is operationally important. Retention drivers in healthcare IT include mission alignment, work-life balance, and meaningful work; compensation is necessary but rarely sufficient.

Performance management for IT staff should align individual goals to portfolio priorities and to operational SLA performance. Annual goal-setting paired with quarterly check-ins is the operational baseline; many organizations have adopted continuous feedback models with formal calibration cycles. Succession planning identifies critical roles and develops named successors at one-year and three-year readiness horizons.

0.47 Communication

Communication competency varies inversely with technical depth in many IT leaders; CPHIMS items often test communication scenarios. The fundamental skill is matching message format and content to the audience.

Executive communication requires concise, decision-oriented framing. A board update on EHR upgrade progress should lead with the status, the decision needed, the cost and schedule variance, and the risk; technical detail belongs in an appendix. Clinical communication requires translation of IT activity into clinical workflow impact. Operational communication should specify what will change, when, and what action the recipient must take. External communication, including regulator-facing communication during breach response, requires precise factual accuracy and legal review.

The communication plan is a project artifact that specifies audience, message type, channel, frequency, and owner for each stakeholder group. A communication plan is not a status report; it defines the structure within which status reports are produced.

0.48 Change Management

Change management is the discipline of guiding individuals, teams, and organizations through transitions. In clinical IT, change management is decisive — a technically successful go-live with poor adoption is operationally a failure.

Three frameworks dominate. The Prosci ADKAR model identifies five sequential outcomes for individual change: Awareness, Desire, Knowledge, Ability, Reinforcement. The framework is diagnostic; if adoption stalls, the model identifies which outcome was not achieved. The Kotter 8-Step framework focuses on organization-level transformation: establish urgency, build a guiding coalition, form a strategic vision, enlist a volunteer army, enable action by removing barriers, generate short-term wins, sustain acceleration, and institute change. Lewin's Change Model offers a simpler three-stage framework: unfreeze, change, refreeze.

Resistance to change is normal and predictable. Common sources include perceived loss (autonomy, prestige, workflow comfort), uncertainty, lack of skill, and lack of consultation. Change management interventions address each source — explicit consultation reduces autonomy concerns, training builds skill, communication reduces uncertainty. Punishing resistance rarely works; understanding the source and addressing it does.

> **Exam Tip**
>
> TCO typically runs 4–7 times vendor list price over a seven-year horizon. When an exam item presents a decision based on list price alone, the correct answer is to complete the TCO analysis.

> **Exam Tip**
>
> ADKAR is sequenced — Awareness must precede Desire, Desire must precede Knowledge, and so on. If a scenario describes a project where users have skills (Knowledge and Ability) but won't use the system, the gap is in Desire or Reinforcement.

> **Key Concept**
> IT governance is decision rights and accountability, not technical decisions. A governance failure manifests as inability to prioritize, not as a specific technology choice.

> **Key Concept**
> Hard savings, soft savings, and avoidance are distinct ROI categories. Finance accepts hard savings without rebuttal; the other two categories require defensible measurement.

> **Key Concept**
> Change management is the predominant determinant of clinical IT success. A technically excellent system with poor adoption fails the organization.

0.49 Chapter Review Questions

Q1. Which COBIT 2019 domain contains governance objectives distinct from management objectives? A) APO B) EDM C) BAI D) DSS **Answer: B** — The Evaluate, Direct, and Monitor (EDM) domain contains COBIT 2019's governance objectives; the APO (Align, Plan, Organize), BAI (Build, Acquire, Implement), DSS (Deliver, Service, Support), and MEA (Monitor, Evaluate, Assess) domains contain management objectives.

Q2. A CFO accepts the IT department's claim of $1.2M in annual savings from a clinical documentation improvement project but requires that the calculation distinguish savings types. Which type does the CFO most readily accept without additional methodology defense? A) Hard savings B) Soft savings C) Cost avoidance D) Productivity gains **Answer: A** — Hard savings are measurable expense reductions or revenue gains visible in the general ledger; finance leaders accept them without additional methodology defense, while soft savings and avoidance require defensible measurement.

Q3. A go-live training program has equipped all users with required system skills, but six weeks post go-live, 30% of users still bypass the new system. Which ADKAR outcome is most likely the gap? A) Awareness B) Knowledge C) Ability D) Reinforcement **Answer: D** — Users have Knowledge and demonstrated Ability but continue to bypass; the missing outcome is Reinforcement, which sustains adoption through accountability, recognition, and removal of bypass options.

Q4. When evaluating vendor proposals for a new oncology information system, which cost dimension represents the largest share of seven-year total cost of ownership for most healthcare IT systems? A) Initial license fee B) Implementation services C) Ongoing support, infrastructure, and integration D) Training **Answer: C** — Ongoing support, infrastructure, and integration costs typically dominate seven-year TCO; initial license is 15–25% of TCO and implementation is another 15–25%.

Q5. A clinical IT project sponsor requests an executive-level status update for the board. Which framing is most appropriate? A) Detailed task-level Gantt chart B) Concise status, decision needed, variance, and risk with technical detail in appendix C) Vendor product roadmap D) Quarterly financial trends since project initiation **Answer: B** — Executive communication leads with status, decision needed, variance, and risk; technical detail belongs in an appendix where it is available but does not impede decision-making.

Testing and Evaluation

Exam Weight: 7% (range 6–9%)

Learning Objectives: - Design and execute test plans across unit, integration, system, user acceptance, performance, and security test layers. - Apply post-implementation evaluation techniques including benefits realization, usability assessment, and outcomes measurement. - Manage defect tracking, severity classification, and resolution workflows. - Apply clinical-safety-focused testing frameworks including HIT Safety Center practices and the SAFER Guides. - Distinguish formative evaluation from summative evaluation and apply each appropriately.

0.50 The Test Pyramid

Software testing in healthcare follows the same pyramid as in other industries. Unit tests verify individual components or functions in isolation. Integration tests verify that components work together correctly across an interface or API. System tests verify end-to-end behavior against requirements. User acceptance tests (UAT) confirm that the system meets the user's needs in a realistic environment. Performance, scalability, and security tests verify non-functional behavior.

Unit and integration testing belong primarily to developers and configuration teams; system and UAT belong primarily to QA and end users. The right ratio is heavily unit-test-weighted (broad base of fast tests) with progressively narrower bands at higher levels. Healthcare environments where integration complexity dominates often invert this ratio, with disproportionately large integration test suites and small unit suites; this is a recognized risk because integration tests are slower, brittler, and more expensive to maintain.

0.51 Test Planning

A test plan documents scope, approach, resources, schedule, and acceptance criteria for testing. The IEEE 829 standard (now superseded by ISO/IEC/IEEE 29119) defines a standard test plan structure. CPHIMS candidates should know the standard test plan sections: introduction, test items, features to be tested, features not to be tested, approach, item pass/fail criteria, suspension and resumption criteria, test deliverables, environmental needs, responsibilities, staffing and training, schedule, risks and contingencies, and approvals.

Test cases should follow a consistent structure: identifier, objective, preconditions, test steps, expected result, actual result, and pass/fail. Traceability from requirement to test case to defect to fix is a Joint Commission and FDA expectation for safety-critical systems.

0.52 User Acceptance Testing

UAT differs from earlier test phases in goal: it confirms that the system meets the user's needs in their environment, not that the system implements the specification. UAT should use real workflows, real data (de-identified where appropriate), and real users. UAT scripts should be developed jointly with end users, not handed down from IT.

UAT scope must include negative and edge cases. A clinical UAT that exercises only the happy path will miss the medication-order conflict that produces an unsafe state at go-live. Common UAT failure modes include insufficient time allocation, IT staff substituting for end users due to schedule pressure, and resolution of UAT defects without re-test.

0.53 Performance, Scalability, and Security Testing

Performance testing measures response time, throughput, and resource consumption under defined load. Load testing applies the expected production load; stress testing pushes beyond the expected load to find the breaking point; endurance testing maintains expected load over an extended period to find slow-developing problems (memory leaks, log file growth, cache exhaustion).

Scalability testing measures the system's ability to handle growth — more users, more transactions, more data. Healthcare scalability has specific patterns: clinic schedules cluster around 8:00 a.m. and 1:00 p.m. starts, generating order entry peaks; surgical post-op periods generate documentation surges; end-of-month finance closes generate batch loads on reporting infrastructure.

Security testing includes vulnerability scanning (automated identification of known vulnerabilities in the deployed stack), penetration testing (skilled attackers simulating real adversary behavior), and code review (static and dynamic analysis of application code). The December 2024 HIPAA Security Rule NPRM proposes annual penetration testing and semi-annual vulnerability scanning at minimum; as of 2026 the NPRM remains a proposal, so candidates should treat these cadences as proposed not finalized while continuing to expect that OCR enforcement practice will reward organizations operating at or above the proposed cadences. CPHIMS candidates should know that vulnerability scanning is automated and broad; penetration testing is human-led, scenario-driven, and targets specific assets.

0.54 Defect Management

Defects discovered during testing should be logged in a defect tracking system with a defined workflow. Defect severity is assigned based on impact (clinical safety, regulatory compliance, operational impact, cosmetic). Severity 1 defects block go-live and require resolution before deployment; lower-severity defects may be deferred to a documented punch list.

Defect classification matters because resource allocation follows it. A common operational error is treating a workflow-flexibility defect (the system requires three clicks where the user expects one) as severity 1 when it is more appropriately classified as a usability defect for a future release. The opposite error — treating a clinical-safety defect as low severity — has caused sentinel events. Defect classification should follow a documented rubric agreed by clinical, operational, and IT leadership.

0.55 Post-Implementation Evaluation

Evaluation continues after go-live. Benefits realization measures whether the projected business benefits actually materialized. A benefits realization plan, developed during analysis, identifies each projected benefit, the measurement method, the baseline, the target, and the measurement schedule. Common healthcare IT benefits include reduced length of stay, increased first-pass denial rate, reduced documentation time, increased throughput, and reduced medication errors.

Benefits realization measurement is difficult because clinical environments are not laboratories. Confounders include concurrent process improvements, seasonal variation, case-mix change, payer policy change, and staff turnover. Defensible benefits realization isolates the IT contribution through statistical controls or by selecting metrics that confounders affect minimally.

Usability evaluation continues post-go-live through System Usability Scale (SUS) surveys, time-on-task measurements, and direct observation. The SUS is a 10-item instrument that produces a 0–100 score; healthcare clinical-software SUS scores tend to fall well below the cross-industry average of 68, reflecting the well-documented usability deficits of legacy EHR products.

0.56 Formative vs Summative Evaluation

Formative evaluation gathers information to improve a system during its development or operation. Summative evaluation measures the system's overall value or effectiveness, typically against the decision to continue, expand, or replace it. Both have a place; an evaluator should know which type they are conducting and design accordingly.

In healthcare IT, formative evaluation drives the iterative optimization that follows initial go-live. Most major EHR implementations remain in active optimization for two to three years post-go-live, with formative evaluation guiding workflow refinement, training redesign, and configuration adjustment.

> **Exam Tip**
>
> UAT is about user needs in the user's environment, not about specification compliance. CPHIMS items test the candidate's recognition that IT staff cannot validly substitute for end users in UAT.

> **Exam Tip**
>
> Vulnerability scanning is automated and broad; penetration testing is human-led, scenario-driven, and asset-targeted. Confusing these is a recurring exam distractor.

> **Key Concept**
>
> The test pyramid favors many unit tests, fewer integration tests, fewer system tests, fewer still UAT tests. Healthcare integration complexity often inverts this and creates operational risk.

> **Key Concept**
>
> Benefits realization must be planned during analysis. A retroactive benefits claim against an unbaselined metric is rarely defensible.

> **Key Concept**
>
> Formative evaluation improves; summative evaluation decides. Match the evaluation type to the decision the evaluation must support.

0.57 Chapter Review Questions

Q1. A health system completes UAT for a new ambulatory EHR. Due to physician scheduling constraints, IT staff executed 60% of the UAT scripts on behalf of clinicians. Which risk does this practice most directly create? A) Increased test execution speed B) UAT defects reflecting IT-staff behavior rather than clinician workflow needs C) Lower defect counts D) Reduced training time **Answer: B** — UAT must reflect user needs in the user's environment; IT-staff substitution produces UAT results that do not reflect clinician workflow needs and increases the risk of post-go-live workflow failures.

Q2. Which type of security test is human-led, scenario-driven, and targets specific assets to simulate adversary behavior? A) Vulnerability scanning B) Penetration testing C) Code review D) Compliance audit **Answer: B** — Penetration testing is human-led, scenario-driven, and targets specific assets; vulnerability scanning is automated and broad.

Q3. A health IT director measures EHR usability using the System Usability Scale six months post-go-live and reports a score of 54. Which interpretation is most accurate? A) Above the cross-industry average of 68 B) Below the cross-industry average of 68 and consistent with reported clinical-software performance C) Indicating immediate need for full system replacement D) Statistically equivalent to industry average and not actionable **Answer: B** — Healthcare clinical-software SUS scores typically fall well below the cross-industry average of 68; a score of 54 is consistent with reported clinical-software performance and signals optimization opportunity, not immediate replacement.

Q4. A project sponsor asks the IT director whether the new revenue cycle system "delivered the projected $4M in annual savings." Which evaluation type is the sponsor requesting? A) Formative B) Summative C) Usability D) Performance **Answer: B** — Summative evaluation measures overall value against a decision; the sponsor's question asks whether projected benefits materialized, which is a summative decision-supporting evaluation.

Q5. Which testing layer should be the broadest base of the test pyramid in a healthy software development practice? A) Unit tests B) Integration tests C) System tests D) User acceptance tests **Answer: A** — The test pyramid favors many fast unit tests at the base with progressively narrower bands at integration, system, and UAT levels; inversions of this shape create operational risk.

0.58 Practice Exam

The following 50 questions cover all seven CPHIMS examination domains in approximate proportional weighting against the 2022 Content Outline (General 16%, Systems Analysis 17%, Systems Design 12%, Selection/Implementation/Support/Maintenance 24%, Privacy and Security 12%, Administration/Leadership/Management 12%, Testing and Evaluation 7%). Treat the practice exam as a timed dress rehearsal: allow yourself 55 minutes total. Mark questions you are uncertain about and review explanations after scoring. A passing score on this practice exam is 35 of 50 correct (70%); strong candidates should target 40 of 50 (80%).

Q1. A 340B-eligible community hospital implements a new pharmacy management system. Which federal program's compliance requirements most directly shape the system's reporting requirements? A) 340B Drug Pricing Program B) Medicare Hospital Outpatient Prospective Payment System C) Drug Supply Chain Security Act D) Section 1115 demonstration **Answer: A** — 340B drug pricing compliance requires the covered entity to prevent diversion to non-eligible patients and to prevent duplicate Medicaid discount, which drives specific tracking and reporting requirements in the pharmacy management system.

Q2. Under TEFCA, which actor operationally designates Qualified Health Information Networks (QHINs)? A) CMS B) The Sequoia Project in its Recognized Coordinating Entity role under contract with ASTP/ONC C) ASTP/ONC directly without an RCE D) State Health Information Exchanges **Answer: B** — ASTP/ONC contracts with The Sequoia Project as the Recognized Coordinating Entity (RCE); it is the Sequoia Project in its RCE role that operationally designates and oversees QHINs. ASTP/ONC retains policy authority but does not designate QHINs directly.

Q3. A hospital's interface engine drops 4% of ADT messages during a sustained vendor outage upstream. The dropped messages are not detected for six hours. Which design improvement most directly addresses this failure mode? A) Increase interface engine CPU B) Implement guaranteed delivery with persistent queueing and end-to-end monitoring C) Switch from HL7 v2 to FHIR D) Replace the interface engine vendor **Answer: B** — Guaranteed delivery with persistent queueing prevents message loss during upstream outage and end-to-end monitoring detects drops promptly; CPU, protocol, and vendor change do not address the root failure.

Q4. Which document is required for disclosure of a Limited Data Set? A) Patient authorization B) Business Associate Agreement C) Data Use Agreement D) Institutional Review Board waiver **Answer: C** — A Data Use Agreement is required under 45 CFR 164.514(e) for disclosure of a Limited Data Set; authorization is not required because an LDS removes specified identifiers.

Q5. A scenario describes 215 distinct duplicate patient records identified for one Mrs. Smith across an EMPI of 1.4M patients. Which root cause is most likely? A) Insufficient EMPI CPU B) Deterministic matching rules with overly tight tolerance for last-name variation C) FHIR API misconfiguration D) Audit log failure **Answer: B** — A high duplicate-per-patient count clustered on one name most directly implicates deterministic matching rules that fail to recognize legitimate name variants (Smith vs. Smithe vs. Smyth vs. Smith-Jones); tuning probabilistic matching or expanding name normalization is the standard response.

Q6. Which MIPS performance category captures EHR-supported quality measure reporting? A) Quality B) Cost C) Improvement Activities D) Promoting Interoperability **Answer: A** — The Quality category captures CQM reporting from certified EHR technology; Promoting Interoperability captures specific interoperability measures distinct from quality.

Q7. A vendor demonstration script includes the scenario "admit a patient with three active allergies, place a conflicting medication order, document the override reason, transfer the patient between units." This scripted scenario is an example of: A) A general happy path demo B) A scenario test that exercises decision support, documentation, and workflow integration C) A penetration test D) A user acceptance test **Answer: B** — The scripted scenario exercises decision support (allergy conflict), documentation (override), and workflow integration (transfer); it is a structured scenario test appropriate for vendor demo, not UAT or pen test.

Q8. An EHR security audit identifies that 47 terminated employees retained active accounts an average of 38 days post-termination. Which IAM lifecycle stage failed? A) Joiner B) Mover C) Leaver D) Authentication **Answer: C** — The Leaver stage of the JML lifecycle failed; terminated employees should have accounts disabled at termination through automated provisioning tied to HR system events.

Q9. Which encryption algorithm represents the operational baseline for data at rest in healthcare environments? A) DES B) 3DES C) AES-256 D) RC4 **Answer: C** — AES-256 is the operational baseline for symmetric encryption at rest; DES, 3DES, and RC4 are deprecated for new deployments.

Q10. A health system's IT steering committee charters the IT portfolio process. Which committee output most directly evidences portfolio management maturity? A) Approval of every IT project request B) Documented rejection of more proposals than approval C) Delegation of all decisions to the CIO D) Quarterly review of vendor contracts only **Answer: B** — Disciplined rejection of more proposals than approval is a measurable governance maturity indicator; approval of every request signals absence of prioritization, not abundance of value.

Q11. An RFP scoring rubric awards 30% weight to technical fit, 25% to financial fit, 20% to vendor stability, 15% to implementation approach, and 10% to references. A vendor scores 90/100 on technical, 70 on financial, 80 on vendor stability, 75 on implementation, and 95 on references. What is the vendor's weighted score? A) 79.5 B) 82.0 C) 81.0 D) 78.5 **Answer: C** — $(90\times0.30) + (70\times0.25) + (80\times0.20) + (75\times0.15) + (95\times0.10) = 27 + 17.5 + 16 + 11.25 + 9.5 = 81.25$, which rounds to 81.

Q12. The HIPAA breach notification clock for individual notification begins at: A) The date the breach occurred B) The date the breach is discovered C) The date legal counsel completes review D) The date the OCR investigation concludes **Answer: B** — The 60-day clock begins at discovery, defined as the first day on which the breach is known or, by exercising reasonable diligence, should have been known.

Q13. A non-functional requirement states "the system shall recover all transactions within 4 hours of a regional power outage." Which non-functional category is this? A) Performance B) Availability and recoverability C) Usability D) Maintainability **Answer: B** — Recovery time after outage is an availability and recoverability requirement, frequently expressed as RTO (Recovery Time Objective).

Q14. Which document standard is required for the CMS Provider Directory API? A) HL7 CDA B) HL7 FHIR R4 with US Core C) X12 5010 D) NCPDP SCRIPT **Answer: B** — The CMS Interoperability and Patient Access Rule requires FHIR R4 with US Core for the Provider Directory API and other regulated APIs.

Q15. A hospital's downtime procedures should be tested at what cadence to satisfy CMS Emergency Preparedness Rule requirements and Joint Commission Information Management expectations? A) An annual full exercise with periodic tabletop and unit-level drills, supplemented based on local risk B) Every five years C) Only after material infrastructure change D) Continuously, in production **Answer: A** — The CMS Emergency Preparedness Rule requires at least annual exercises; the Joint Commission EM and IM standards do not impose a quarterly cadence. Annual full exercises supplemented by periodic tabletops and unit-level drills, with additional cadence determined by local risk assessment, is the operational baseline; some organizations test more frequently for risk-based reasons.

Q16. A clinician requests a printed copy of the EHR's allergy alert configuration before signing off on a new release. Which artifact best supports this request? A) Source code review B) Configuration documentation derived from the system's clinical decision support build C) Vendor marketing collateral D) Implementation Gantt chart **Answer: B** — Configuration documentation derived from the actual clinical decision support build documents the rules and overrides as deployed; vendor collateral and project schedules do not capture configuration state.

Q17. A Lean Six Sigma DMAIC project targets ED throughput. Which project phase produces the Cause-and-Effect (Ishikawa) diagram? A) Define B) Measure C) Analyze D) Improve **Answer: C** — The Analyze phase identifies and validates root causes; Ishikawa (fishbone) diagrams are standard Analyze-phase tools.

Q18. Under HIPAA, which entity directly handles enforcement of the Privacy Rule and the Security Rule? A) Centers for Medicare and Medicaid Services B) Office for Civil Rights C) Office of the National Coordinator D) Federal Trade Commission **Answer: B** — The HHS Office for Civil Rights (OCR) enforces the Privacy, Security, and Breach Notification Rules; CMS enforces Transactions and Code Sets and Provider Identifier rules.

Q19. A facility's enterprise data warehouse is structured with conformed dimensions for patient, provider, and time. Which dimensional modeling concept does "conformed" describe? A) Dimensions are normalized to third normal form B) Dimensions are shared across multiple fact tables with identical structure and content C) Dimensions have surrogate keys D) Dimensions are denormalized **Answer: B** — Conformed dimensions are shared across multiple fact tables with identical structure and content, enabling cross-process analysis; this is a foundational Kimball methodology concept.

Q20. Which severity classification should be assigned to a defect where the EHR allows medication orders to be placed for a discharged patient, with no warning? A) Severity 1 (blocker) B) Severity 2 (major) C) Severity 3 (minor) D) Severity 4 (cosmetic) **Answer: A** — A defect that allows medication orders against a discharged patient is a clinical safety issue and should be classified Severity 1 (blocker); resolution is required before deployment.

Q21. Which framework provides ten knowledge areas for managing projects and is the dominant general project management body of knowledge? A) ITIL v4 B) PMBOK C) COBIT 2019 D) TOGAF **Answer: B** — PMBOK identifies ten knowledge areas (integration, scope, schedule, cost, quality, resource, communications, risk, procurement, stakeholder) and is the dominant general project management framework.

Q22. A health information exchange uses the IHE XCA profile for cross-community exchange. XCA stands for: A) Cross-Enterprise Audit B) Cross-Community Access C) Cross-Channel Authentication D) Cross-Coverage Adjustment **Answer: B** — XCA is Cross-Community Access, the IHE profile for retrieving documents from multiple communities.

Q23. Which physical safeguard category under the HIPAA Security Rule includes workstation security policies? A) Facility access controls B) Workstation use and workstation security C) Device and media controls D) Contingency operations **Answer: B** — Workstation Use (164.310(b)) and Workstation Security (164.310(c)) are distinct standards within the physical safeguards category.

Q24. A hospital's CIO presents the board with a five-year IT investment plan totaling $48M. Which financial concept best supports comparison of investment options with different time profiles? A) Net Present Value B) Internal Rate of Return C) Payback Period D) Return on Investment **Answer: A** — Net Present Value accounts for the time value of money across the full investment horizon and is the preferred basis for comparing options with different time profiles.

Q25. A clinical decision support governance committee approves the addition of a sepsis early-warning rule based on a predictive model in a certified Health IT product. Which post-implementation activity is required by the HTI-1 DSI criterion and by responsible governance? A) Annual review of rule firing rate, clinical action rate, and continued conformance to the developer's published source attributes and IRMP B) One-time validation only at deployment C) Code-level review of the rule logic D) Replacement of the rule every 12 months regardless of performance **Answer: A** — Predictive DSI requires ongoing review of firing rate, clinical action rate, and conformance to the developer's published source attributes and Intervention Risk Management Practice (IRMP); one-time validation is insufficient under HTI-1 and under responsible deployment-side governance.

Q26. Under TEFCA, the QHIN-to-QHIN exchange supports which six formally named Exchange Purposes as defined in the Common Agreement and SOPs? A) Treatment, Payment, Health Care Operations, Public Health, Government Benefits Determination, Individual Access Services B) Treatment, Payment, Operations only C) Research and Public Health only D) Treatment and Individual Access only **Answer: A** — The Common Agreement and TEFCA Standard Operating Procedures define six Exchange Purposes by their formal names: Treatment, Payment, Health Care Operations (two words), Public Health, Government Benefits Determination, and Individual Access Services.

Q27. A health system's HCAHPS scores have stagnated. Which IT investment is most likely to move the metric? A) Increased server capacity B) Communication-supporting tools (rounding apps, patient portals, real-time discharge education) C) Enhanced infrastructure monitoring D) Vendor-managed help desk **Answer: B** — HCAHPS measures patient experience including communication; IT investments that support communication and patient engagement most directly affect the metric.

Q28. Which artifact documents the trace from requirements through design, code, and tests? A) Traceability matrix B) Project charter C) Gantt chart D) Vendor SLA **Answer: A** — A requirements traceability matrix maps each requirement to its sources, design artifacts, code, and test cases, supporting impact analysis and compliance.

Q29. A workflow analysis identifies that nurses paper-document medication administration during a 90-second EHR latency window and then back-enter the data after the system responds. The dominant defect type is: A) Network latency B) Workflow misalignment with system performance characteristics C) User training gap D) Hardware capacity insufficiency **Answer: B** — The 90-second latency is unacceptable for active medication administration workflow; the defect is workflow misalignment with system performance, and the response is either workflow redesign, performance improvement, or both.

Q30. Which incident management metric measures the time from incident detection to incident resolution? A) Mean Time Between Failures B) Mean Time to Restore C) Mean Time to Resolution D) Mean Time to Acknowledge **Answer: C** — Mean Time to Resolution measures the elapsed time from incident detection to permanent fix; Mean Time to Restore measures service restoration which may precede full resolution.

Q31. A FHIR API implementation must support which authentication framework to comply with SMART App Launch 2.1? A) Basic Auth B) OAuth 2.0 with FHIR-specific scopes C) API Key in URL parameter D) HTTP Digest **Answer: B** — SMART App Launch 2.1 requires OAuth 2.0 with FHIR-specific scopes; Basic Auth, URL keys, and Digest are not compliant.

Q32. A senior CIO reviews a 240-page RFP response. Which review approach is most consistent with sound vendor selection practice? A) Personally read the entire document B) Delegate review to a structured evaluation team scoring against the published rubric C) Skim the executive summary D) Forward to legal counsel for sole review **Answer: B** — Structured evaluation teams scoring against the published rubric defend the selection decision, distribute the work appropriately, and reduce single-reviewer bias.

Q33. Which clinical workflow is most likely to depend on real-time HL7 v2 ADT messaging? A) Annual financial reconciliation B) Hospital census and bed management C) Quarterly quality reporting D) End-of-year tax reporting **Answer: B** — Hospital census and bed management depend on real-time admission, discharge, and transfer events; HL7 v2 ADT messaging is the operational backbone.

Q34. A health system performs an IT risk assessment using a 5×5 likelihood × impact scoring matrix. A risk with likelihood 2 (low) and impact 2 (low) produces a raw risk score of 4. Which risk response is most likely appropriate? A) Accept and document B) Avoid through scope reduction C) Transfer through insurance D) Mitigate with high-cost controls **Answer: A** — A low-likelihood, low-impact risk with a score of 4 sits unambiguously in the "accept and document" band of standard healthcare risk matrices. Acceptance is reserved for low-likelihood AND low-impact combinations; higher-frequency operational risks (even with low single-event impact) typically warrant mitigation or monitoring rather than pure acceptance.

Q35. Under the Privacy Rule, which disclosure to a family member requires patient agreement (which may be inferred from the circumstances)? A) Disclosure to law enforcement under a warrant B) Disclosure of relevant information to family members involved in care C) Disclosure to a public health authority D) Disclosure of psychotherapy notes **Answer: B** — Disclosures to family members involved in the patient's care are permitted with the patient's agreement, which may be inferred from circumstances under 45 CFR 164.510(b).

Q36. A new revenue cycle system's projected benefits include a 2-percentage-point reduction in first-pass denial rate. Which baseline measurement should be captured before go-live? A) Average length of stay B) Current first-pass denial rate over a defined period C) Patient satisfaction score D) Coding accuracy by DRG **Answer: B** — Benefits realization requires a baseline measurement of the specific metric the benefit targets; only the current first-pass denial rate provides a defensible baseline.

Q37. Which structured query language standard underpins most enterprise reporting from clinical data warehouses? A) NoSQL B) ANSI SQL C) GraphQL D) XPath **Answer: B** — ANSI SQL is the dominant standard for relational data warehouse querying; NoSQL, GraphQL, and XPath serve different domains.

Q38. A patient requests electronic access to their lab results through the patient portal. Under the ONC Information Blocking Rule, which response by the provider is most consistent with compliance? A) Decline pending a fee analysis B) Provide access through the available API and patient portal C) Require an in-person visit before release D) Provide a printed copy only **Answer: B** — The Information Blocking Rule requires providers to make EHI accessible through available APIs and portals; declining, requiring an in-person visit, or providing only print would be likely-to-interfere practices absent an applicable exception.

Q39. A clinical informatics team observes that physicians override 88% of drug-drug interaction alerts. The dominant problem is most likely: A) Excessive false-positive alert rate (low specificity) B) Physician malpractice C) Vendor configuration bug D) Insufficient training **Answer: A** — An 88% override rate is the classic alert fatigue signature, indicating excessive false positives and low alert specificity; the response is to tune the rule set, not to retrain or discipline clinicians.

Q40. A health information exchange uses a single auto-link threshold in its identity matching algorithm — records above the threshold are linked automatically, records below enter a manual review queue. The HIE lowers this threshold from 0.92 to 0.88. Under this single-threshold design, the expected effects are: A) Increased automatic links and increased manual queue B) Increased automatic links and decreased manual queue C) Decreased automatic links and increased manual queue D) Decreased automatic links and decreased manual queue **Answer: B** — In a single-threshold design, lowering the threshold accepts more matches automatically (increased auto-links) and reduces the manual review queue, while increasing false-positive risk. (In a two-threshold design with separate auto-link, manual-review, and auto-reject bands, the effect on the manual queue depends on how the bands move; candidates should read scenario stems carefully for the design specified.)

Q41. A nurse manager requests an EHR change that would let nurses chart vital signs in advance of taking them. Which response is most appropriate? A) Implement the change to reduce charting time B) Decline due to clinical safety and data integrity concerns and offer to redesign workflow to reduce charting friction C) Refer to vendor for evaluation D) Implement with a manager override **Answer: B** — Charting in advance of observation creates safety risk (false documentation of unperformed assessment) and data integrity risk; the appropriate response is to decline the change and address the underlying workflow friction.

Q42. Which COBIT 2019 design factor most directly captures regulatory environment differences across organizations? A) Enterprise strategy B) Compliance requirements C) IT-related issues D) Threat landscape **Answer: B** — Compliance requirements is the COBIT 2019 design factor capturing regulatory environment differences; the other factors capture strategy, current issues, and threat respectively.

Q43. A clinical informatics director plans a SAFER Guides self-assessment. Which approach satisfies the assessment's intent? A) IT department completes the assessment unilaterally B) Multidisciplinary team including clinical, IT, and quality completes the assessment C) External vendor completes the assessment D) Single physician completes the assessment **Answer: B** — The SAFER Guides are designed for multidisciplinary self-assessment by clinical, IT, and quality leaders; single-discipline completion does not satisfy the assessment's intent.

Q44. Which acronym in the HIPAA breach risk assessment refers to the four factors a covered entity must consider? A) Confidentiality, Integrity, Availability, Auditability B) Nature/extent of PHI, person who used/received it, whether actually acquired/viewed, mitigation C) Probability, Impact, Detection, Response D) Threat, Vulnerability, Asset, Control **Answer: B** — The Omnibus Rule's four-factor breach risk assessment considers the nature and extent of PHI, the unauthorized person who used or received it, whether the PHI was actually acquired or viewed, and the extent to which the risk has been mitigated.

Q45. A vendor offers a "free upgrade" to a major new EHR release. Which financial analysis correctly characterizes the offer? A) Genuinely free with no organizational cost B) Free of vendor license cost but substantial organizational cost for implementation, training, validation, and downtime C) Free with full vendor support included D) Free with mandatory cash rebate **Answer: B** — License-free upgrades carry substantial organizational cost in implementation, training, validation, and downtime; total upgrade cost may exceed the original license value.

Q46. Which clinical workflow standard governs the message content for laboratory orders and results? A) HL7 v2 ORM (order) and ORU (result) B) DICOM C) NCPDP SCRIPT D) X12 837 **Answer: A** — HL7 v2 ORM (order) and ORU (result) are the standard messages for laboratory order and result exchange; DICOM is imaging, NCPDP is e-prescribing, X12 837 is claims.

Q47. A patient access representative pulls a celebrity's record on her shift. The representative authenticated with valid credentials and her role's RBAC permissions allowed the access, so authorization did not prevent it. Internal audit later flagged the access through audit-log review and user behavior analytics. Which combination of safeguards actually detected the violation? A) Authentication and physical access only B) Audit controls and analytics monitoring C) Encryption only D) Network firewall **Answer: B** — When authentication is valid and authorization permits the access at the role level, neither acts as a detective control. Audit controls (164.312(b)) recorded the access event, and the user behavior analytics platform flagged the anomaly; together they constitute the detective safeguards. Authorization in this scenario is the failed preventive safeguard, not a detective one.

Q48. Which standard underpins claims submission from a healthcare provider to a payer? A) HL7 v2.5.1 B) X12 837 C) DICOM D) NCPDP SCRIPT **Answer: B** — X12 837 is the claims submission standard; the corresponding remittance standard is X12 835. HIPAA Transactions and Code Sets Rule mandates these standards for covered transactions.

Q49. A health system uses a SOC 2 Type II report from a vendor. Which assurance does the report provide? A) Vendor financial stability B) Vendor controls over security, availability, processing integrity, confidentiality, and privacy as designed and operating over a defined period C) HIPAA compliance certification D) ONC certification **Answer: B** — SOC 2 Type II reports cover trust services criteria (security, availability, processing integrity, confidentiality, privacy) as designed and operating over a defined period (typically 6–12 months); SOC 2 is not a HIPAA or ONC certification.

Q50. A CIO is asked to recommend whether the organization should adopt a cloud-first IT strategy. Which analysis most directly supports a defensible recommendation? A) Vendor marketing material review B) Multi-criteria analysis covering TCO, security, compliance, latency, integration, and exit costs across a defined planning horizon C) Survey of peer CIOs D) Single-vendor sandbox trial **Answer: B** — Strategic IT decisions require multi-criteria analysis across the dimensions that meaningfully differ between options over a defined horizon; vendor material, peer surveys, and single-vendor trials are inputs but not sufficient bases for the decision.

Exam Quick Reference

Exam structure: 115 questions (100 scored + 15 pre-test), 120 minutes (2-hour testing window), scaled score 600 to pass on a 400–800 scale. Computer-based delivery in Pearson VUE testing centers or via Pearson VUE OnVUE remote proctoring. Verify the current window length and delivery options in the HIMSS Candidate Handbook in effect on the date of registration.

Domain weights (2022 Content Outline, in force for 2026 administrations): General 16% • Systems Analysis 17% • Systems Design 12% • Systems Selection/Implementation/Support/Maintenance 24% • Privacy and Security 12% • Administration, Leadership, Management 12% • Testing and Evaluation 7%. Total = 100%.

Pacing target: roughly one minute per question (115 questions in 120 minutes); reserve 5–10 minutes for flagged-item review.

Key federal regulations and where to find them: - HIPAA Privacy Rule: 45 CFR 160 + 164 Subparts A and E - HIPAA Security Rule: 45 CFR 160 + 164 Subparts A and C (administrative 164.308, physical 164.310, technical 164.312) - HIPAA Breach Notification Rule: 45 CFR 164.400–414 - ONC Cures Act Final Rule (Information Blocking): 45 CFR Part 171, eight exceptions (Security Exception at 171.203) - ONC HTI-1 Final Rule: 45 CFR Part 170 (DSI criterion at 170.315(b)(11)) - CMS Interoperability and Patient Access Rule: 45 CFR Parts 422, 431, 438, 457, 482, 485 - CMS Interoperability and Prior Authorization Final Rule (January 2024): extends FHIR-based exchange to PA workflows - OIG Information Blocking Civil Money Penalty Rule (September 2023): penalties up to $1M per violation for developers/HINs - CMS Provider Disincentives Rule (July 2024): program-specific disincentives for providers found to have committed information blocking

Information Blocking Exceptions (eight, all at 45 CFR Part 171): Preventing Harm, Privacy, Security (171.203), Infeasibility, Health IT Performance, Content and Manner, Fees, Licensing.

Required FHIR baseline: HL7 FHIR Release 4 with US Core Implementation Guide. Current SMART specifications: SMART App Launch 2.1 (May 2024) for user-facing apps; SMART Backend Services for system-to-system flows.

HTI-1 DSI essentials: Two classes — evidence-based and predictive. Source attribute disclosures required for both, expanded list for predictive. Intervention Risk Management Practice (IRMP) summary must be publicly available. Source: 45 CFR 170.315(b)(11).

USCDI status: USCDI v3 is the current certified Health IT floor (via HTI-1); v4 published July 2023, v5 published July 2024 — both in the pipeline for future rulemaking.

Standards quick map: HL7 v2 (real-time messaging) • HL7 CDA (documents) • HL7 FHIR (APIs) • DICOM (imaging) • SNOMED CT (clinical terms) • LOINC (labs/document codes) • RxNorm (medications) • ICD-10-CM (diagnoses, including SDOH Z codes Z55–Z65) • ICD-10-PCS (inpatient procedures) • CPT (outpatient procedures) • NCPDP SCRIPT (e-prescribing) • X12 837/835/270/271/276/277 (claims, remittance, eligibility, claim status).

TEFCA Exchange Purposes (six, formal SOP-defined names): Treatment, Payment, Health Care Operations, Public Health, Government Benefits Determination, Individual Access Services. RCE = The Sequoia Project under contract with ASTP/ONC.

Project management EVM formulas: SV = EV − PV • CV = EV − AC • SPI = EV/PV • CPI = EV/AC • Values <1.0 are behind plan.

HIPAA breach notification clock: 60 days from discovery for individual notice; immediate notice to OCR and prominent media for breaches affecting ≥500 residents of a state or jurisdiction; annual to OCR for <500.

HIPAA civil money penalty tiers: Tier 1 (lack of knowledge) • Tier 2 (reasonable cause, not willful neglect) • Tier 3 (willful neglect, corrected ≤30 days) • Tier 4 (willful neglect, not corrected). Each tier has per-violation min/max and per-year cap; HHS adjusts annually for inflation. Verify current Federal Register figures near exam time.

Security Rule safeguard examples: - Administrative: risk analysis, workforce training, security incident procedures, contingency plans, sanction policy - Physical: facility access controls, workstation use and security, device and media controls - Technical: access control, audit controls, integrity, person/entity authentication, transmission security

NIST SP 800-63B AAL terminology: AAL1 (single factor) • AAL2 (two factors; practical clinical baseline; may include phishing-vulnerable factors like SMS OTP) • AAL3 (hardware-bound, phishing-resistant; recommended for high-risk roles).

MIPS performance categories: Quality • Cost • Improvement Activities • Promoting Interoperability. Annual weights set in the CY-year QPP Final Rule (CMS typically publishes in November of the preceding year). Verify CY 2026 weights in the CY 2026 QPP Final Rule near exam time.

MoSCoW prioritization: Must (non-negotiable) • Should (high value, deferrable) • Could (nice to have) • Won't (this release).

ITIL processes commonly tested: Incident Management (restore service) • Problem Management (root cause) • Change Management (controlled deployment) • Release Management (coordinated release) • Service Request Management (standard requests).

Change management ADKAR sequence: Awareness □ Desire □ Knowledge □ Ability □ Reinforcement.

NIST Cybersecurity Framework 2.0 Functions (six): Govern (new in 2.0) • Identify • Protect • Detect • Respond • Recover.

Glossary

Accountable Care Organization (ACO): A group of healthcare providers that voluntarily accepts responsibility for the cost and quality of care for an attributed population, typically under Medicare Shared Savings Program contracts.

Addressable Implementation Specification: Under HIPAA Security Rule, a specification that the covered entity must implement, document a reasonable alternative that achieves the objective, or document why neither is reasonable. Not optional.

Alternative Payment Model (APM): A payment approach that gives providers incentives or risk for delivering high-quality care; Advanced APMs qualify for the QPP track separate from MIPS.

ASTP/ONC: Assistant Secretary for Technology Policy / Office of the National Coordinator for Health Information Technology — the post-2024 name of the HHS office responsible for health IT certification, interoperability rulemaking, and TEFCA policy.

ATNA (Audit Trail and Node Authentication): IHE profile standardizing audit event format and transport across systems.

Authentication: Establishing who a user is.

Authenticator Assurance Level (AAL): NIST SP 800-63B classification of authentication strength; AAL1 (single factor), AAL2 (two factors; practical clinical baseline), AAL3 (hardware-bound and phishing-resistant; for high-risk roles).

Authorization: Establishing what an authenticated user may do.

Breach (HIPAA): The acquisition, access, use, or disclosure of PHI in a manner not permitted by the Privacy Rule that compromises the security or privacy of the PHI.

Business Associate (BA): A person or entity that performs functions or activities on behalf of a covered entity that involve the use or disclosure of PHI; bound by a Business Associate Agreement and directly subject to many Security Rule requirements after HITECH.

CDA (Clinical Document Architecture): HL7 document exchange standard; CCD (Continuity of Care Document) is a commonly tested CDA template.

CMS Provider Disincentives Rule (2024): CMS final rule applying program-specific disincentives (loss of Promoting Interoperability credit, MSSP disqualification, etc.) to providers found by OIG to have committed information blocking.

COBIT 2019: Governance and management framework for enterprise IT; separates governance objectives (EDM) from management objectives (APO, BAI, DSS, MEA).

Computerized Physician Order Entry (CPOE): Electronic entry of clinical orders by the ordering practitioner.

Conformed Dimension: A dimension shared across multiple fact tables with identical structure and content, enabling cross-process analysis.

Covered Entity (CE): Under HIPAA, a health plan, healthcare clearinghouse, or healthcare provider that conducts certain electronic transactions.

Critical Access Hospital (CAH): A Medicare-designated rural hospital with up to 25 beds and special cost-based reimbursement.

CSF 2.0 (NIST Cybersecurity Framework 2.0): February 2024 update to the NIST framework; adds Govern as a sixth Function alongside Identify, Protect, Detect, Respond, Recover.

Data Use Agreement (DUA): Required document for disclosure of a Limited Data Set under HIPAA Privacy Rule.

Decision Support Intervention (DSI): ONC certification criterion at 45 CFR 170.315(b)(11) (HTI-1 Final Rule) governing both evidence-based and predictive (including AI/ML) clinical decision support, with source attribute disclosure and Intervention Risk Management Practice requirements.

De-identification: Removing identifiers from PHI to convert it to non-PHI; two methods are Safe Harbor (18 identifier types) and Expert Determination.

EHR Certification (ONC): Voluntary certification of health IT against ASTP/ONC certification criteria; required to participate in some federal programs and to support information-blocking-compliant functions.

EMPI (Enterprise Master Patient Index): A system that uniquely identifies patients across multiple source systems within an enterprise.

Encryption: The conversion of data into a form that cannot be readily understood without a key.

EV (Earned Value): The value of work completed to date, measured against the project baseline.

FHIR (Fast Healthcare Interoperability Resources): HL7 API-based exchange standard; Release 4 with US Core is the required US baseline.

Formative Evaluation: Evaluation that gathers information to improve a system during development or operation.

Gap Analysis: Comparison of current to desired state across defined dimensions to identify gaps requiring closure.

HIE (Health Information Exchange): The electronic sharing of health information among organizations; also refers to the organizations that facilitate such sharing.

HIPAA (Health Insurance Portability and Accountability Act): Federal statute enacted 1996, the foundation of US health information regulation.

HITECH (Health Information Technology for Economic and Clinical Health Act): 2009 statute that created the Meaningful Use program and substantially strengthened HIPAA enforcement; introduced the four-tier civil money penalty structure.

HTI-1 Final Rule: ONC Health Data, Technology, and Interoperability Final Rule (December 2023), introducing the DSI certification criterion, updating the USCDI floor to v3, and adding Insights Condition and Maintenance of Certification requirements.

HTI-2 NPRM: ONC Health Data, Technology, and Interoperability NPRM (August 2024), proposing public health, payer, patient engagement, and additional API certification criteria; not finalized as of late 2025.

ICD-10-CM: International Classification of Diseases, 10th Revision, Clinical Modification, used for diagnosis coding; includes SDOH Z codes Z55–Z65.

ICD-10-PCS: International Classification of Diseases, 10th Revision, Procedure Coding System, used for inpatient procedure coding.

Incident (ITIL): Any event that causes or may cause a disruption to a service.

Information Blocking: Under 45 CFR Part 171, a practice by a covered actor that is likely to interfere with the access, exchange, or use of EHI; eight exceptions are defined (Security Exception at 171.203).

Integration Engine: A software platform that routes, transforms, and queues messages between healthcare systems.

Intervention Risk Management Practice (IRMP): Developer-side governance documenting risk analysis, mitigation, and post-deployment monitoring of a DSI; publicly summarized as required by HTI-1.

ITIL v4: Service management framework dominant in healthcare IT operations.

Joint Commission: Independent accrediting body recognized by CMS as a deeming authority for hospitals and other healthcare organizations.

LOINC (Logical Observation Identifiers Names and Codes): Terminology for lab observations and document type codes, maintained by Regenstrief Institute.

MIPS (Merit-based Incentive Payment System): One of two QPP tracks; performance scored across Quality, Cost, Improvement Activities, and Promoting Interoperability categories; weights set annually in the CY-year QPP Final Rule.

MoSCoW Prioritization: Requirements prioritization framework: Must, Should, Could, Won't.

OCR (Office for Civil Rights): HHS enforcement office for HIPAA Privacy, Security, and Breach Notification Rules.

OMOP (Observational Medical Outcomes Partnership) Common Data Model: Standardized data model for cross-institution research and analytics, governed by OHDSI.

PCCP (Predetermined Change Control Plan): FDA guidance (finalized December 2024) for AI/ML-enabled SaMD allowing manufacturers to make specified, pre-authorized post-market modifications without new pre-market submissions.

Person-Centered Care: Approach to care that respects the patient's preferences, needs, and values.

PHI (Protected Health Information): Individually identifiable health information held or transmitted by a covered entity or business associate.

Penetration Testing: Human-led, scenario-driven security testing that simulates adversary behavior against specific assets.

PGHD (Patient-Generated Health Data): Data captured by or for the patient outside a clinical encounter, including wearables and home monitoring data; foundational to RPM and RTM billing categories.

Problem (ITIL): The cause of one or more incidents.

Promoting Interoperability (PI): Successor to Meaningful Use; MIPS category and parallel program for hospitals (Medicare Promoting Interoperability Program).

Qualified Health Information Network (QHIN): A TEFCA-designated network-of-networks participant; designated and overseen by The Sequoia Project as RCE under contract with ASTP/ONC.

Recognized Coordinating Entity (RCE): Under TEFCA, the contractor that designates and oversees QHINs and publishes the Common Agreement and SOPs; The Sequoia Project holds this role under contract with ASTP/ONC.

Risk Analysis (HIPAA): Accurate and thorough assessment of potential risks and vulnerabilities to ePHI required under 45 CFR 164.308(a)(1)(ii)(A).

Risk Register: Document tracking identified risks, current state, planned responses, and residual risk.

RPM (Remote Patient Monitoring): Medicare-reimbursable remote physiologic monitoring service category (CPT 99453–99458) requiring device qualification, minimum data days, and clinical review time.

RPO (Recovery Point Objective): Maximum acceptable data loss measured as a time interval before disruption.

RTO (Recovery Time Objective): Maximum acceptable time to restore service after disruption.

Ryan Haight Act: 2008 federal statute requiring an in-person evaluation before controlled substance prescribing; in-person requirement waived by DEA on a series of extensions since the COVID-19 PHE.

SAFER Guides: ASTP/ONC self-assessment tools for safe EHR practices across nine domains.

SDOH (Social Determinants of Health): Non-clinical factors affecting health outcomes; captured in USCDI SDOH elements, ICD-10-CM Z codes (Z55–Z65), and the CMS Health Equity Index in MIPS.

SMART App Launch 2.1: Current widely-deployed version of the SMART specification for user-facing third-party FHIR app authentication and authorization (OAuth 2.0).

SMART Backend Services: SMART specification for system-to-system FHIR exchange using JWS-signed client assertions; used for CMS Bulk Data exports and Da Vinci flows.

SNOMED CT: Clinical terminology governed by SNOMED International.

SOC 2 Type II: Vendor assurance report covering trust services criteria as designed and operating over a defined period.

SPI (Schedule Performance Index): EV/PV; values <1.0 indicate schedule behind plan.

Sentinel Event: Joint Commission–defined patient safety event resulting in death, permanent harm, or severe temporary harm.

Star Schema: Dimensional data model with a central fact table surrounded by dimension tables.

Summative Evaluation: Evaluation that measures overall value or effectiveness against a continue/expand/replace decision.

TEFCA (Trusted Exchange Framework and Common Agreement): Nationwide exchange framework under ASTP/ONC; QHINs operate under a Common Agreement administered by The Sequoia Project as RCE; six Exchange Purposes (Treatment, Payment, Health Care Operations, Public Health, Government Benefits Determination, Individual Access Services).

TCO (Total Cost of Ownership): Acquisition plus implementation, training, ongoing operations, integration, and decommissioning costs over economic life.

USCDI (United States Core Data for Interoperability): ASTP/ONC's standardized floor data set for certified Health IT; v3 is the current floor (via HTI-1); v4 (July 2023) and v5 (July 2024) are in the version pipeline.

US Core Implementation Guide: US-specific FHIR profiles required by CMS Interoperability rules.

User Acceptance Testing (UAT): Confirmation that the system meets user needs in the user's environment.

Vulnerability Scanning: Automated identification of known vulnerabilities in deployed systems.

Work Breakdown Structure (WBS): Hierarchical decomposition of a project into deliverables and work packages.

X12 837: Claims submission standard mandated by HIPAA Transactions and Code Sets Rule.

Study Schedule

The 8-week schedule allocates 10–12 hours per week for 80–100 total hours and assumes the candidate has some current professional exposure to healthcare IT. The 4-week schedule allocates 15–20 hours per week for 60–80 total hours and assumes substantial recent experience across multiple domains. Both schedules end with a full timed practice exam followed by targeted weak-area review and a one-day rest before the exam.

8-Week Schedule

Week 1: General domain orientation. Read Chapter 1 twice. Build a one-page personal regulatory reference covering HIPAA, HITECH, the ONC Cures Act Final Rule, the HTI-1 Final Rule, the CMS Interoperability and Prior Authorization Rules, and TEFCA. Take Chapter 1 review questions cold; review explanations for misses and correct guesses. Read ASTP/ONC's information blocking exceptions one-pager, the HTI-1 DSI summary, and the CMS Interoperability and Prior Authorization Rule overview. Verify the CY 2026 MIPS category weights in the QPP Final Rule. Time investment: 10 hours.

Week 2: Systems Analysis. Read Chapter 2. Build practice swimlane and BPMN diagrams for a workflow you know in your current role. Take Chapter 2 review questions and conduct a 30-minute self-debrief on requirements categories (business, functional, non-functional). Time investment: 10 hours.

Week 3: Systems Design. Read Chapter 3. Sketch an n-tier, microservices, and integration-engine-mediated architecture for the same hypothetical hospital. Map ten exam-relevant standards to their domains from memory. Write a one-page summary of the HTI-1 DSI source attribute and IRMP requirements and the FDA PCCP framework for AI/ML SaMD. Take Chapter 3 review questions. Time investment: 10 hours.

Week 4: Systems Selection, Implementation, Support, Maintenance, Part 1. Read Chapter 4 sections through "Project Management Discipline." Practice five EVM calculations until SPI, CPI, SV, and CV are automatic. Take half of Chapter 4 review questions. Time investment: 12 hours.

Week 5: Systems Selection, Implementation, Support, Maintenance, Part 2. Complete Chapter 4 and review the support tier and decommissioning sections. Build a one-page incident vs. problem vs. known error reference. Complete Chapter 4 review questions. Time investment: 10 hours.

Week 6: Privacy and Security. Read Chapter 5 twice. Memorize the eight Information Blocking exceptions (with the Security Exception at 45 CFR 171.203), the three Security Rule safeguard categories with three examples each, the 60-day breach notification clock mechanics, the four HIPAA penalty tiers, and the NIST AAL2 vs AAL3 distinction. Look up the current Federal Register HIPAA penalty inflation adjustment. Take Chapter 5 review questions. Time investment: 12 hours.

Week 7: Administration, Leadership, Management + Testing and Evaluation. Read Chapters 6 and 7. Build a one-page ADKAR-and-Kotter reference and a one-page test pyramid reference. Take Chapters 6 and 7 review questions. Time investment: 12 hours.

Week 8: Full practice exam and targeted review. Take the 50-question practice exam under timed conditions (55 minutes). Score by domain and identify the two weakest domains. Spend three days reviewing those domains using the relevant chapters and external resources (ASTP/ONC, CMS, OCR guidance documents). Day before exam: light review of Appendix A only; rest. Time investment: 14 hours.

4-Week Schedule

Week 1: General + Systems Analysis + Systems Design. Read Chapters 1, 2, and 3. Take all chapter review questions and review explanations. Build the personal regulatory reference and standards map. Verify CY 2026 MIPS weights in the QPP Final Rule. Time investment: 20 hours.

Week 2: Systems Selection/Implementation/Support/Maintenance. Read Chapter 4 twice. Practice EVM calculations. Build incident/problem/change reference. Complete chapter review. Time investment: 18 hours.

Week 3: Privacy and Security + Administration, Leadership, Management + Testing and Evaluation. Read Chapters 5, 6, and 7. Memorize eight Information Blocking exceptions, the HIPAA four-tier penalty structure, and NIST AAL distinctions. Complete all chapter review questions. Time investment: 20 hours.

Week 4: Full practice exam and targeted review. Take the 50-question practice exam under timed conditions. Score by domain, review the two weakest domains for three days. Day before exam: review Appendix A only; rest. Time investment: 14 hours.

Both schedules assume that the candidate takes notes on misses and correct guesses, reviews Appendix B vocabulary in 15-minute daily increments throughout, and resists the temptation to substitute new study resources for the disciplined work in the chapter material. Candidates who take the practice exam more than once should expect score inflation on the second attempt; the most informative score is the cold first attempt.

A final note on exam day. Sleep, hydration, and a routine breakfast outperform any last-minute cramming. Bring two forms of ID, arrive 30 minutes early at the Pearson VUE center (or complete the OnVUE system check 24 hours in advance for remote delivery), and trust your preparation. The CPHIMS exam rewards disciplined, broad knowledge across the seven domains; no single domain dominates, and no single answer trick will save a candidate who has not done the work. Candidates who follow the schedule, score above 70% on the practice exam, and arrive rested pass at well above the historical first-attempt pass rate.

Best of luck on exam day, and congratulations in advance on joining the more than 7,500 healthcare IT professionals worldwide who hold the CPHIMS credential.

Enterprise Architecture, IT Governance, and Strategic Planning

Exam Weight: Approximately 12–16 percent (Administration and Leadership domain)

.1 Learning Objectives

After completing this chapter, the candidate will be able to:

- Distinguish the major enterprise architecture frameworks (TOGAF and Zachman) and explain how the business, data, application, and technology layers organize an integrated delivery network's information assets.
- Construct an IT strategic plan that aligns with organizational strategy through an application portfolio assessment, capability roadmap, and explicit linkage to enterprise goals.
- Apply IT governance frameworks (COBIT and ITIL) and describe the decision rights vested in an IT steering committee, a clinical governance council, and an architecture review board.
- Evaluate IT investments using total cost of ownership, return on investment, net present value, and payback, and structure capital versus operating budgets and benefits-realization measurement at a strategic level.
- Develop enterprise data governance through stewardship, master data management, and a single source of truth, and formulate build-versus-buy, best-of-breed-versus-single-vendor, and technical-debt rationalization strategies.

.2 Enterprise Architecture Frameworks and the Four Architecture Layers

Enterprise architecture (EA) is the discipline of describing an organization's structure, processes, information, and technology as a coherent whole so that change can be planned rather than improvised. For a CPHIMS candidate operating at the senior level, EA is the connective tissue between clinical strategy and technical execution: it ensures that a decision to expand ambulatory services, adopt value-based contracts, or consolidate a merged hospital's systems is translated into deliberate changes across applications, data, and infrastructure rather than a patchwork of point solutions.

The two frameworks the exam expects you to recognize are TOGAF and Zachman. **The Open Group Architecture Framework (TOGAF)** is a process-and-method framework. Its centerpiece is the **Architecture Development Method (ADM)**, a cyclical sequence of phases—Architecture Vision, Business Architecture, Information Systems Architecture (which splits into data and application), Technology Architecture, Opportunities and Solutions, Migration Planning, Implementation Governance, and Architecture Change Management—anchored by Requirements Management at the center. TOGAF also defines an **Architecture Repository** and an **Architecture Content Framework** of deliverables (artifacts and building blocks) that let an organization treat architecture as a managed, reusable asset rather than a set of one-off diagrams.

The **Zachman Framework**, by contrast, is a taxonomy, not a process. It is a two-dimensional matrix whose columns ask the six primitive interrogatives—**What (data), How (function), Where (network), Who (people), When (time), and Why (motivation)**—and whose rows describe perspectives from the executive (scope/contextual) down through business management, architect, engineer, and technician to the operating enterprise. Zachman tells you which questions must be answered and from whose viewpoint; it does not tell you how to proceed. Many health systems use the two together: Zachman to classify and audit completeness, TOGAF's ADM to sequence the work.

Both frameworks resolve into four conventional **architecture layers**. The **business architecture** layer captures the organization's strategy, governance, clinical and revenue-cycle processes, and the capabilities the enterprise must possess (for example, "schedule a patient," "reconcile medications," "adjudicate a claim"). The **data architecture** layer describes the logical and physical structure of information assets—patient demographics, clinical observations, financial transactions—along with their relationships, semantics, and lineage. The **application architecture** layer describes the application portfolio and the interactions among systems: the electronic health record (EHR), the laboratory information system, the enterprise resource planning (ERP) suite, the integration engine, and the analytics platform, together with the integration patterns that connect them. The **technology architecture** layer (also called infrastructure architecture) describes the hardware, networks, cloud services, operating systems, and platform services that host everything above. The discipline of EA is to keep these four layers consistent so that a change in a business capability propagates predictably into data, application, and technology decisions.

> **Key Concept**
>
> Enterprise architecture is not a one-time diagram. It is a living governance practice that maintains traceability from business strategy through the data, application, and technology layers so that every system investment can be justified by a business capability it enables. The CPHIMS leader uses EA to prevent the accumulation of redundant, undocumented, and orphaned systems.

.3 IT Strategic Planning and Alignment with Organizational Strategy

The **IT strategic plan** is the document and process by which IT leadership commits its scarce resources—capital, people, and attention—to the goals of the enterprise over a multi-year horizon, typically three to five years with annual refresh. The single most important property of a credible IT strategic plan is **alignment**: every major initiative should trace to an organizational objective such as improving quality outcomes, growing market share, reducing cost per case, succeeding under value-based contracts, or improving the patient and clinician experience. Strategic alignment is the central theme of the **Strategic Alignment Model**, which holds that IT and business strategies must align both *strategically* (high-level direction) and *operationally* (infrastructure and processes), and in both directions—IT enabling the business and the business shaping IT.

A senior IT strategic plan typically contains a current-state assessment, a future-state vision, a gap analysis, and a sequenced roadmap with resourcing and financial implications. The current-state assessment rests on an **application portfolio assessment**, often visualized using the **TIME model—Tolerate, Invest, Migrate, Eliminate**—or a comparable two-axis grid that plots each application's *business value* against its *technical fitness*. Applications that are high value and technically sound warrant continued investment; those that are high value but technically fragile are candidates for migration or replacement; those low in both dimensions are candidates for elimination. This disciplined scoring of the portfolio is what separates a strategic plan from a wish list, because it forces explicit decommissioning decisions rather than perpetual accretion.

From the portfolio assessment flows the **capability roadmap**, a time-phased view of which business capabilities the organization will build, enhance, or retire and when. A roadmap is organized around capabilities and outcomes rather than projects, which keeps it stable even as individual projects start, slip, or are reprioritized. The roadmap is paired with a financial forecast that distinguishes the run-the-business spend (keeping current systems operating) from the grow-and-transform spend (new capabilities). A common senior-level diagnostic is the ratio of "keep the lights on" spending to discretionary investment; an organization spending the overwhelming majority of its IT budget simply to operate has little capacity to execute strategy and must rationalize before it can transform.

> **Exam Tip**
>
> When a question describes an IT initiative and asks how to justify or prioritize it, the best answer almost always references explicit linkage to an organizational strategic goal, not the technology's sophistication. The exam consistently rewards business–IT alignment over technical novelty.

.4 IT Governance Frameworks: COBIT, ITIL, and the Governing Bodies

IT governance is the system of decision rights and accountabilities that ensures IT investments deliver value and that IT-related risk is managed. Governance answers *who decides* and *who is accountable*; management answers *who does the work*. The exam expects fluency in two complementary frameworks.

COBIT (Control Objectives for Information and Related Technologies), maintained by ISACA, is a governance-and-management framework. Its current edition, COBIT 2019, draws a sharp line between **gover-**

nance (the **Evaluate, Direct, and Monitor**, or **EDM**, objectives that belong to the board and executive level) and **management** (objectives grouped as Align/Plan/Organize, Build/Acquire/Implement, Deliver/Service/Support, and Monitor/Evaluate/Assess). COBIT is the framework of choice for demonstrating that IT is controlled, that risk is managed, and that performance is measured against enterprise goals; it is frequently the reference point for audits and regulatory assurance.

ITIL (Information Technology Infrastructure Library) is a framework for **IT service management (ITSM)**—the operational practices that deliver and support IT services through their lifecycle. ITIL 4 organizes work around the **Service Value System** and the **Service Value Chain** and defines management practices such as **incident management** (restoring service quickly), **problem management** (eliminating root causes), **change enablement** (controlling changes through a change advisory board), **service request management**, **service level management** (codified in service level agreements), and **configuration management** (maintaining the configuration management database, or CMDB). Where COBIT governs and assures, ITIL delivers and supports; mature organizations use COBIT as the governance umbrella and ITIL as the operational discipline beneath it.

Frameworks are inert without governing bodies. The **IT steering committee** is the senior cross-functional body—typically chaired by an executive sponsor and including the CIO, CMIO, CNIO, CFO, and operational and clinical leaders—that sets IT priorities, approves the portfolio, allocates funding, and arbitrates competing demands. Its essential function is portfolio-level prioritization: deciding which of many worthy initiatives the organization will actually fund and sequence. Distinct from it, a **clinical governance council** (or clinical informatics committee) owns clinical content and workflow decisions: order sets, clinical decision support rules, documentation standards, and the clinical impact of system changes. Keeping clinical governance separate from the steering committee ensures that frontline clinical judgment, not IT convenience, governs the clinical use of systems. A third body, the **data governance council**, is discussed below.

.5 Portfolio, Program, and Project Management with Demand Management

At enterprise scale, IT work must be managed as a portfolio, not a collection of independent projects. **Project portfolio management (PPM)**—and at the largest scale **enterprise portfolio management**—is the centralized practice of selecting, prioritizing, and balancing the entire set of IT investments to maximize value within capacity and risk constraints. The hierarchy the exam expects you to distinguish is precise: a **project** is a temporary endeavor producing a defined deliverable; a **program** is a coordinated group of related projects managed together to achieve benefits not available from managing them individually (an EHR optimization program might encompass projects for documentation redesign, decision support, and reporting); and a **portfolio** is the complete set of programs, projects, and operational investments selected to advance strategy. PMI's standards and the **Program Management Office (PMO)** or **Enterprise PMO** provide the methods and the oversight body.

The front door to the portfolio is **demand management**, also called **intake**. A disciplined intake process requires every request—whether for a new application, an enhancement, or an integration—to be submitted, scored against consistent criteria (strategic alignment, financial return, risk, regulatory necessity, and resource demand), and prioritized through governance before resources are committed. Without intake discipline, IT is captured by whoever shouts loudest or has the most senior sponsor, and the portfolio drifts from strategy. The intake process also performs an essential triage between **mandatory** work (regulatory and safety obligations that must be funded), **keep-the-lights-on** work, and **discretionary** investment, ensuring the organization funds its obligations before its aspirations. Capacity planning—matching the prioritized demand against the realistic supply of analyst, developer, and clinical-informaticist hours—is what converts a prioritized list into an executable plan.

> **Key Concept**
>
> Demand management (intake) is the governance control that prevents the IT portfolio from being driven by political pressure rather than strategic value. A consistent, scored intake process is the single most effective tool a senior IT leader has for protecting capacity for the work that matters most.

.6 Benefits Realization, Total Cost of Ownership, and Investment Valuation

Approving an investment is not the same as obtaining its value. **Benefits realization** is the disciplined process of defining the expected benefits of an investment before approval, assigning ownership for delivering them, measuring whether they materialize after implementation, and holding the organization accountable for the gap. HIMSS has long emphasized that the great majority of value from health IT comes not from the technology itself but from the process redesign and adoption around it; a benefits-realization framework therefore tracks **outcome measures** (reduced length of stay, fewer adverse drug events, improved charge capture, reduced denial rates) rather than activity measures (number of systems installed). The discipline requires a **baseline** measurement taken before go-live, target benefits with named owners, and post-implementation measurement against the baseline. The recurring senior lesson is that benefits realization is an operational and clinical responsibility, not an IT deliverable; IT enables the capability, but operational leaders own the outcome.

Sound investment decisions begin with **total cost of ownership (TCO)**, which captures the full multi-year cost of an investment—not merely the acquisition price but implementation, integration, interfaces, training, ongoing licensing or subscription, infrastructure, support staffing, and eventual decommissioning. A persistent error in health IT is to compare alternatives on license price alone; a "cheaper" best-of-breed system can carry far higher TCO once interface development, additional staffing, and upgrade burden are counted. TCO is the denominator against which value must be weighed.

For the value side, the exam expects you to distinguish the standard capital-budgeting measures. **Return on investment (ROI)** expresses net benefit as a percentage of cost and is intuitive but ignores timing. **Net present value (NPV)** discounts all future cash flows—costs and benefits—back to present dollars using a discount rate; a positive NPV indicates an investment that creates value after accounting for the time value of money, and NPV is generally the most rigorous single measure for comparing investments of different sizes and time profiles. **Internal rate of return (IRR)** is the discount rate at which NPV equals zero, useful for comparison against a hurdle rate. **Payback period** is the time required to recover the initial outlay; it is simple and communicates risk exposure but ignores everything after payback and the time value of money. A senior leader presents a business case using several measures together—TCO for the full cost picture, NPV for rigorous value, and payback for an intuitive risk read—because no single number captures the whole decision.

.7 IT Financial Management: Capital versus Operating Budgets

Strategic financial management of IT turns on the distinction between capital and operating expenditure, because it shapes both accounting and decision-making. **Capital expenditure (CapEx)** funds assets with multi-year useful life—data-center hardware, perpetual software licenses, major implementations—that are recorded on the balance sheet and depreciated over time. **Operating expenditure (OpEx)** funds recurring costs—subscriptions, cloud consumption, support contracts, maintenance, and salaries—expensed in the period incurred. The migration of health IT from on-premise systems toward **software-as-a-service (SaaS)** and cloud platforms has shifted spending decisively from CapEx toward OpEx, which improves flexibility and reduces large up-front outlays but converts predictable depreciation into variable, consumption-based expense that must be actively managed (a discipline often called cloud financial management or FinOps). The senior IT leader must construct a budget that funds three categories simultaneously: mandatory and regulatory obligations, run-the-business operations, and strategic growth—and must defend that budget to a CFO in the language of TCO, depreciation, and cash-flow timing rather than feature lists.

> **Exam Tip**
>
> Know the CapEx/OpEx distinction cold. A perpetual license and on-premise servers are CapEx (capitalized and depreciated); a SaaS subscription and cloud consumption are OpEx (expensed as incurred). Questions frequently test whether a cloud migration shifts spending from capital to operating budgets—it does.

Beyond the annual budget, mature organizations practice **IT financial management** as an ongoing discipline: showback or chargeback that attributes IT cost to the business units that consume it (making demand visible and creating accountability), benchmarking IT spend as a percentage of operating revenue against peer health systems, and managing the run-versus-transform ratio deliberately over time. Showback informs consumers of what their demand costs without billing them; chargeback actually allocates the cost to their budgets and is the stronger demand-control mechanism but requires the cultural and accounting maturity to administer fairly.

.8 Enterprise Data Governance: Stewardship, MDM, and a Single Source of Truth

As health systems consolidate and as analytics and artificial intelligence become central to clinical and financial strategy, **enterprise data governance** rises to a board-level concern. Data governance is the framework of policies, roles, and processes that ensures data is accurate, consistent, secure, and fit for use across the enterprise. Its governing body is the **data governance council**, which sets data policy and arbitrates definitions; its operational backbone is **data stewardship**. A **data steward** is an individual—usually embedded in a business or clinical domain rather than in IT—accountable for the quality, definitions, and appropriate use of a specific data domain such as patient identity, provider data, or revenue-cycle data. The steward owns the meaning of the data; IT owns the systems that store it.

The technical centerpiece of enterprise data governance is **master data management (MDM)**: the discipline and tooling that create and maintain authoritative, deduplicated records for the core entities the enterprise shares across systems—patients, providers, locations, and items. In healthcare, the canonical MDM problem is patient identity. An **enterprise master patient index (EMPI)** reconciles patient records across the EHR, registration, laboratory, radiology, and billing systems so that the organization can assert a **single source of truth** for who a patient is, preventing duplicate records and the patient-safety hazards of a fragmented identity. Provider master data, managed similarly, underpins credentialing, scheduling, billing, and directory accuracy. The strategic objective of MDM is to replace many conflicting versions of a core entity with one governed, authoritative version that every downstream system trusts.

A single source of truth extends beyond master entities to metrics and definitions. When the chief financial officer and the chief medical officer present different figures for the same readmission rate because their systems define the numerator and denominator differently, the failure is one of data governance, not technology. Enterprise data governance establishes a **business glossary** of agreed definitions and a governed analytics layer—often an enterprise data warehouse or lakehouse—so the organization argues about strategy rather than about whose number is right.

.9 Standards, Architecture Review Boards, and Investment Discipline

To keep the four architecture layers coherent over time, the enterprise needs standing bodies that enforce consistency at the moment decisions are made. The **architecture review board (ARB)**, sometimes called a technical review board, reviews proposed solutions against approved standards, reference architectures, and the target-state architecture before money is committed. The ARB enforces **standards**—approved integration patterns (such as HL7 v2 messaging and **HL7 FHIR** APIs), approved platforms, security baselines, and interoperability requirements—and is the gatekeeper that prevents well-intentioned projects from introducing redundant or non-conforming technology. A **standards committee** may maintain the catalog of approved standards that the ARB enforces. Embedding architecture review in the intake and approval workflow is how an organization operationalizes EA rather than leaving it as documentation that projects ignore.

These bodies are where two recurring strategic choices are adjudicated. The first is **build versus buy**. Building custom software offers a tailored fit and potential competitive differentiation but carries high development cost, ongoing maintenance burden, and key-person risk; buying commercial software offers vendor support, regulatory updates, and a shared upgrade path but constrains the organization to the vendor's model. The senior default in healthcare is to buy commodity capability and reserve building for genuine differentiation, because a health system's competitive advantage rarely lies in writing its own registration or billing software.

The second is **best-of-breed versus single-vendor (suite) strategy**. A **best-of-breed** approach selects the strongest individual application in each domain—the best laboratory system, the best radiology system—accepting the cost and fragility of integrating them. A **single-vendor** or **integrated-suite** approach (an EHR vendor providing registration, clinical, revenue-cycle, and ancillary modules) trades some functional depth for native integration, a single data model, unified support, and lower integration TCO. The prevailing trend in the United States has been consolidation toward integrated suites, driven by the integration cost and patient-safety risk of stitching together many systems; but the right answer is contingent on the organization's size, existing investments, and where functional gaps would create unacceptable clinical or financial risk. The architecture review board is precisely the body that should weigh these trade-offs against the target architecture rather than letting them be decided system by system.

.10 Managing Technical Debt and System Rationalization

The accumulated cost of expedient past decisions—aging platforms, unsupported software versions, brittle custom interfaces, duplicated systems acquired through mergers, and undocumented workarounds—is **technical debt**. Like financial debt, technical debt carries interest: every year it persists, it raises operating cost, slows new development, increases security and compliance risk (unsupported software cannot be patched), and reduces reliability. A senior IT leader treats technical debt as a managed liability with a deliberate paydown plan, not as an embarrassment to be hidden, and quantifies it where possible so that the steering committee can weigh debt reduction against new-capability investment.

The principal remedy is **application rationalization (or system rationalization)**: the systematic review of the application portfolio to consolidate redundant systems, retire those that are low-value or unsupported, and standardize on a smaller, governed set of platforms. Rationalization is the natural and ongoing output of the application portfolio assessment described earlier; the TIME or value-versus-fitness scoring identifies elimination and migration candidates, and rationalization executes their decommissioning. Mergers and acquisitions make this urgent, because each acquisition typically arrives with its own overlapping systems, and the integrated organization cannot afford to operate three of everything. Done well, rationalization reduces TCO, shrinks the attack surface, simplifies the data and integration landscape, and frees the run-the-business budget that funds transformation—closing the loop back to the IT strategic plan with which this chapter began. The senior discipline is to make rationalization a permanent governance practice rather than a periodic crisis response, so the portfolio is continuously pruned in step with strategy.

.11 Chapter 8 Review Questions

Q1. A health system is documenting its enterprise architecture and wants a method that sequences architecture work through defined, iterative phases from vision through migration planning and change management. Which framework's Architecture Development Method best meets this need?

A) The Zachman Framework
B) TOGAF
C) COBIT 2019
D) ITIL 4

Answer: B — TOGAF provides the Architecture Development Method (ADM), an iterative, phased *process* for developing architecture. Zachman is a taxonomy (a classification matrix), not a process method; COBIT governs IT, and ITIL manages IT services. Because the requirement is for a sequenced method, TOGAF's ADM is correct.

Q2. During capital budget planning, the CIO proposes replacing on-premise servers and perpetual software licenses with a cloud-hosted SaaS platform billed by subscription. From a financial-management standpoint, what is the primary effect of this change?

A) It shifts spending from operating expenditure to capital expenditure
B) It shifts spending from capital expenditure to operating expenditure
C) It eliminates total cost of ownership considerations
D) It converts depreciation into a one-time capital charge

Answer: B — Perpetual licenses and on-premise hardware are capitalized assets (CapEx) that are depreciated over their useful life. A SaaS subscription and cloud consumption are recurring costs expensed as incurred (OpEx). The migration therefore shifts spending from CapEx to OpEx. TCO remains highly relevant, and the change moves away from depreciation rather than converting it into a one-time charge.

Q3. Two executives present conflicting 30-day readmission rates because their respective systems define the measure differently. Which enterprise capability most directly addresses this problem?

A) Master data management of the patient index
B) Service level management under ITIL
C) Enterprise data governance, including a governed business glossary and single source of truth
D) Architecture review board approval of integration standards

Answer: C — The failure is one of inconsistent metric definitions across the enterprise, which is the domain of data governance: a business glossary of agreed definitions and a governed analytics layer establish a single source of truth for shared metrics. MDM addresses master entity identity (such as patients), not metric definitions; ITIL service management and the ARB address service operations and architecture standards, not analytic definitions.

Q4. An IT steering committee must choose among many worthy project requests with insufficient capacity to fund them all. Which governance practice provides the most effective, consistent control over which work is funded?

A) Benefits realization measurement after go-live
B) A scored demand management (intake) process tied to strategic criteria
C) Total cost of ownership analysis of each vendor
D) An ITIL change advisory board review

Answer: B — Demand management (intake) requires every request to be submitted and scored against consistent strategic, financial, risk, and resource criteria before resources are committed, protecting capacity for the highest-value work and preventing political prioritization. Benefits realization measures value after the fact; TCO informs a single business case; and the change advisory board controls production changes, not portfolio funding decisions.

Q5. A merged health system operates three overlapping laboratory systems and several unsupported legacy applications, raising operating cost and security risk. Which senior IT discipline most directly addresses this accumulated condition?

A) Best-of-breed system selection
B) Application rationalization to reduce technical debt
C) Benefits realization framework deployment
D) Capability roadmap publication

Answer: B — The redundant and unsupported systems represent technical debt, and the discipline of systematically consolidating redundant systems and retiring low-value or unsupported ones is application (system) rationalization. Best-of-breed selection would tend to add specialized systems rather than reduce them; benefits realization measures value of investments; and a capability roadmap plans future capabilities but does not itself execute the decommissioning that rationalization performs.

Advanced Data Analytics, Business Intelligence, and Population Health Informatics

Exam Weight: Approximately 10–14 percent (Systems and Analytics)

.12 Learning Objectives

After completing this chapter, the candidate will be able to:

- Architect and govern an enterprise analytics stack—data warehouse, lakehouse, data marts, ETL/ELT, semantic layer, and business-intelligence tooling—and position an organization along the descriptive-to-prescriptive analytics maturity model.
- Establish enterprise data governance, master data management, and data-quality programs that make analytics trustworthy, and govern the lifecycle of clinical machine-learning models, including validation, drift detection, and bias monitoring.
- Design population health informatics capabilities—risk stratification, registries, care-gap analytics, and social-determinants-of-health integration—using health-information-exchange-fed views.
- Operationalize value-based care analytics, including total cost of care, electronic clinical quality measures (eCQMs), and attribution logic.
- Apply real-world-data and interoperability-enabled analytics (FHIR Bulk Data, USCDI) while protecting privacy through de-identification, limited data sets, and HIPAA-compliant data handling.

.13 The Enterprise Analytics Stack

Senior health-IT leaders are accountable not for individual reports but for the **analytics platform**—the layered architecture that converts transactional data into governed, reusable, decision-grade information. The foundational pattern remains the **enterprise data warehouse (EDW)**: a subject-oriented, integrated, time-variant, nonvolatile repository optimized for query and analysis rather than transaction processing. In healthcare, EDWs typically organize data into conformed **dimensions** (patient, provider, encounter, location, date) and **fact tables** (charges, lab results, claims lines) using dimensional modeling—Kimball-style star and snowflake schemas—so that disparate source systems share a common analytic grammar.

The contemporary alternative and complement is the **data lakehouse**, which merges the low-cost, schema-on-read flexibility of a **data lake** (raw files in object storage—Parquet, ORC, Avro) with the transactional reliability, schema enforcement, and performance of a warehouse. Open table formats such as **Delta Lake**, **Apache Iceberg**, and **Apache Hudi** provide ACID transactions, time travel, and schema evolution directly on lake storage, allowing a single copy of data to serve SQL analytics, machine learning, and streaming. For a CPHIMS-level leader, the lakehouse decision is governance and cost as much as technology: it reduces data duplication and supports unstructured clinical data (notes, images, waveforms) that traditional EDWs handled poorly.

Downstream, **data marts** expose curated, department-scoped slices—oncology, revenue cycle, quality—so consumers query a performant, access-controlled subset rather than the full warehouse. Movement into and across these structures occurs through **ETL** (extract, transform, load) or the increasingly favored **ELT** (extract, load, transform). ELT lands raw data first and transforms inside the warehouse/lakehouse engine, exploiting cloud elastic compute and enabling reproducible, version-controlled transformation pipelines (the pattern popularized by tools such as **dbt**). The distinction matters for governance: ELT preserves raw lineage for audit and re-processing, whereas classic ETL discards intermediate states.

The **semantic layer** is the often-underappreciated control point. It defines business metrics—"30-day readmission rate," "total cost of care," "ED throughput"—once, centrally, with agreed definitions, joins, and filters, so that every dashboard and self-service query computes them identically. Without a semantic layer, the organization suffers **metric drift**: two executives quote different readmission numbers because their tools encoded different denominators. Modern **BI tools** (Tableau, Power BI, Qlik, Looker, and embedded analytics platforms) consume this layer to render **clinical and operational dashboards**, paginated reports, and ad hoc exploration.

Key Concept

The semantic layer—not the BI tool—is where "one version of the truth" actually lives. A CPHIMS leader who allows each department to define core measures inside individual dashboards has guaranteed irreconcilable numbers and eroded executive trust in analytics.

.14 The Analytics Maturity Model

A widely used framework positions analytic capability along a continuum of escalating value and difficulty. **Descriptive analytics** answers *what happened*—counts, trends, scorecards, regulatory reports. **Diagnostic analytics** answers *why it happened* through drill-down, root-cause analysis, cohorting, and correlation (for example, decomposing a length-of-stay increase by service line and payer). **Predictive analytics** answers *what is likely to happen*—readmission risk, sepsis onset, no-show probability—using statistical and machine-learning models. **Prescriptive analytics** answers *what should we do*, recommending or automating actions through optimization, simulation, and decision logic (for instance, optimal OR scheduling or staffing under constraints).

Maturity is not merely about owning algorithms; it is organizational. Higher maturity requires data quality, governance, a skilled analytics workforce, integration of insight into workflow (not just dashboards), and a culture that acts on evidence. HIMSS itself operationalizes this through the **Adoption Model for Analytics Maturity (AMAM)**, a staged (0–7) assessment that evaluates an organization's analytic governance, data content, and the extent to which analytics drive care transformation and prescriptive action. Senior leaders use AMAM-style models to benchmark, justify investment, and sequence capability-building—recognizing that prescriptive aspirations are worthless atop poor descriptive foundations.

The leadership implication of the model is sequencing discipline. Organizations routinely over-invest in headline predictive and prescriptive projects while their descriptive and diagnostic layers remain unreliable—producing impressive proofs of concept that never reach durable production because the underlying data cannot be trusted, the workforce cannot interpret outputs, or the operational workflow has no place to receive a recommendation. A defensible analytics roadmap therefore advances on multiple fronts in parallel: foundational data governance and quality, workforce competency, and workflow integration must mature alongside algorithmic ambition. The CPHIMS-level leader is judged not by the sophistication of the most advanced model in the portfolio but by the *floor*—the reliability of routine descriptive reporting that the entire enterprise consumes daily, and the proportion of insight that is actually embedded in care and operational workflows rather than stranded in dashboards no one opens.

Exam Tip

Order matters. The exam may present a scenario and ask which analytics tier it represents. Map verbs: *what happened* = descriptive, *why* = diagnostic, *what will happen* = predictive, *what should we do / what's optimal* = prescriptive. An "alert recommending an intervention" is prescriptive even if a predictive model underlies it.

.15 Enterprise Data Governance, MDM, and Data Quality

Analytics inherits the trustworthiness of its inputs, so the senior leader's first investment is **enterprise data governance:** the accountability framework defining who can take what action, on which data, under what circumstances, using what methods. Effective governance establishes **data stewards** (business owners accountable for definitions and quality of a domain), **data custodians** (technical caretakers), a **data governance council**, and a **business glossary** of authoritative definitions. Governance also owns the **data catalog** and **data lineage**—the documented flow of each data element from source system through transformation to report—which is essential for impact analysis, audit, and regulatory defensibility.

Master data management (MDM) is governance made operational for the entities that recur everywhere. In healthcare the canonical examples are the **enterprise master patient index (EMPI)**, which resolves a single patient across registration systems despite name variants and identifier collisions, and the **provider master / provider data management**, which reconciles clinician identity across credentialing, scheduling, billing, and directory systems. MDM employs deterministic and **probabilistic matching** to link records, manages

golden records (the surviving best-of-breed attribute set), and governs duplicate resolution and merge/unmerge workflows. For analytics, a weak EMPI silently fractures a patient's history across multiple identities, corrupting longitudinal measures, utilization, and risk scores.

Data quality management programs measure and remediate along recognized dimensions: **completeness, accuracy, consistency, timeliness, validity, and uniqueness**. Mature programs do not chase quality reactively; they instrument pipelines with automated **data quality rules** and **data observability** (freshness checks, volume anomalies, schema-change detection, null-rate monitoring) so that a broken interface or an upstream change is caught before it poisons a board report. They also distinguish **data quality** (fitness of the data) from **information quality** (fitness of the delivered insight in context). For clinical quality and value-based programs, regulators increasingly scrutinize data provenance and quality, making a documented data-quality program a compliance asset, not merely an engineering nicety.

.16 Dashboards, Self-Service BI, and Governance of Insight

Clinical and operational dashboards translate the stack into action. **Operational dashboards** are real-time or near-real-time and drive immediate decisions—ED tracking boards, OR utilization, bed capacity, command-center situational awareness. **Tactical and strategic dashboards** aggregate over longer windows for managers and executives—quality scorecards, throughput trends, financial performance against budget. Good design discipline applies: a small set of relevant, validated metrics; clear targets and thresholds; avoidance of chart-junk; and explicit metric definitions visible to the user. Dashboards should drive to action; a "wall of numbers" that no one can act upon is a governance failure, not a design preference.

The strategic tension at senior level is **self-service BI governance**. Democratizing analytics—letting nurse managers, service-line directors, and quality analysts build their own views—accelerates insight and relieves the central analytics team. But ungoverned self-service breeds the very metric drift the semantic layer exists to prevent, alongside security exposure and conflicting "shadow" reports. The mature posture is **governed self-service**: a curated, certified semantic layer and certified datasets; tiered content (IT-certified vs. user-generated, clearly badged); role-based access aligned to minimum necessary; a content lifecycle (promotion, certification, retirement of stale dashboards); and a stewardship model where central analytics owns shared metrics while business users compose presentations atop them. The leader's job is to enable autonomy without surrendering the single version of the truth.

.17 Predictive Modeling and MLOps at the Management Level

As organizations push into predictive and prescriptive tiers, the CPHIMS-level concern shifts from building models to **governing the model lifecycle**—the discipline known as **MLOps (machine-learning operations)**. The lifecycle spans problem framing, data preparation and **feature engineering**, model development, **validation**, deployment, monitoring, and retirement. Leaders are accountable for each gate, not the mathematics.

Validation must address performance *and* generalizability. Discrimination is measured by metrics such as the **AUROC (area under the receiver operating characteristic curve)**; calibration—whether predicted probabilities match observed rates—is assessed separately, because a model can rank patients well yet systematically over- or under-state absolute risk. A defensible program validates on a **held-out** and ideally a **temporally or externally separate** cohort, recognizing that a model trained on one site's population may fail on another (the well-documented hazard with vendor-supplied predictive tools).

After deployment, **monitoring** is continuous, not one-time. **Data drift** (the input distribution shifts—new coding practices, a new lab analyzer, a pandemic) and **concept drift** (the relationship between inputs and outcome changes) degrade performance silently; the program must instrument input distributions, output distributions, and, where feasible, realized outcomes. Equally mandatory is **bias and fairness monitoring**: evaluating performance and error rates across demographic subgroups (race, ethnicity, sex, age, payer, language) because models trained on historically inequitable data—or using proxies such as prior cost for "health need"—can encode and amplify disparities. The leader ensures fairness metrics are defined, measured, and reviewed by governance.

This is the province of **algorithmic governance / clinical algorithm governance**: a multidisciplinary committee (clinical, informatics, data science, compliance, equity, legal) that reviews intended use, validation evidence, equity assessment, integration into workflow, override and feedback mechanisms, and a re-validation cadence. The committee maintains an **inventory of deployed clinical algorithms**—including embedded EHR models and third-party tools—with documented intended use and performance. This aligns with the regulatory and transparency direction of the era: the ONC **HTI-1** rule's requirements for **predictive decision support intervention (DSI)** transparency obligate certified health IT to surface "source attributes" (intended use, training data characteristics, validation, fairness, and how the model was developed) so that organizations can evaluate algorithms for **fairness, appropriateness, validity, effectiveness, and safety (FAVES).** A senior leader treats every clinical algorithm as a governed clinical intervention with a lifecycle, not a static feature.

> **Key Concept**
> A predictive model is never "done." Without monitoring for drift and subgroup bias plus a defined re-validation cadence, a once-validated clinical algorithm becomes an unmonitored medical decision-maker—an unacceptable safety and equity exposure. Governance of the model lifecycle, not model accuracy at launch, is the CPHIMS deliverable.

.18 Population Health Informatics

Population health informatics applies these capabilities to defined populations rather than individual encounters. Its workhorse is **risk stratification**: classifying members by likelihood of adverse outcomes or high utilization so that finite care-management resources concentrate where they yield most benefit. Stratification draws on claims, clinical data, pharmacy, utilization, and increasingly social data, often using **risk-adjustment and grouping methodologies—HCC (Hierarchical Condition Categories)** for CMS risk adjustment, **CDPS**, the **ACG System**, **ERG/DxCG**, and the **LACE** index for readmission risk—alongside custom predictive models. The leader ensures the chosen methodology fits the program (CMS-HCC for Medicare Advantage and ACO risk capture; commercial groupers elsewhere) and that capture is complete and compliant, since under-coding suppresses appropriate risk scores and revenue.

Registries—disease, condition, and procedure registries (diabetes, heart failure, oncology, immunization)—provide the denominator-and-numerator backbone for population management and quality reporting. **Care-gap analytics** then identifies members overdue for evidence-based services (A1c testing, cancer screening, vaccinations, retinopathy exams) and routes actionable worklists to care teams—closing the loop from analytics to intervention. The senior concern is that gaps are *actionable and current*: gaps built on stale or incomplete data erode clinician trust and waste outreach.

Social determinants of health (SDOH) data—housing instability, food insecurity, transportation, financial strain—materially affect outcomes and cost, and population health programs increasingly ingest them. Standards now support this: **Z-codes (ICD-10-CM Z55–Z65)** capture social risk in coded form; the **Gravity Project** defines value sets and FHIR profiles for SDOH; and **USCDI v4 and later** include SDOH data classes (problems/assessments, goals, interventions). Leaders must govern SDOH data carefully—it is sensitive, often self-reported and incomplete, and prone to bias if used naively in algorithms—while integrating it to target whole-person interventions.

HIE-fed population views complete the picture. A single organization sees only the care it delivers; a member's full utilization—out-of-network ED visits, specialist care, admissions elsewhere—arrives through **health information exchanges** and national frameworks. **Admit/Discharge/Transfer (ADT)** event notifications (mandated for many hospitals under CMS Conditions of Participation) feed near-real-time alerts that drive transitional-care and care-management workflows; a discharge notification from an out-of-network hospital is often the single most actionable signal a care-management team receives, triggering the 48-to-72-hour post-discharge outreach that demonstrably reduces avoidable readmissions. The maturing **TEFCA (Trusted Exchange Framework and Common Agreement)** and its **Qualified Health Information Networks (QHINs)** expand nationwide query and exchange, increasingly supporting population-level and treatment use cases beyond the document-centric exchange of earlier eras. A population health platform that ignores external utilization systematically under-counts risk and misses the highest-leverage intervention moments. The senior leader's task is to fuse these external feeds with internal data through the EMPI—so that an external ADT reliably matches the right internal patient record—and to convert raw event streams into governed, deduplicated, and prioritized worklists rather than an undifferentiated flood of alerts that overwhelms care teams and trains them to ignore the channel.

.19 Value-Based Care Analytics

Value-based care converts population insight into financial accountability, and its analytics are exacting. **Total cost of care (TCOC)** aggregates all spending for an attributed population over a period—often **per member per month (PMPM)**—across inpatient, outpatient, professional, pharmacy, and post-acute settings, frequently normalized through **risk adjustment** so that performance comparisons account for population acuity. TCOC analytics underpin shared-savings and capitation arrangements and demand reliable, complete claims plus accurate attribution.

Attribution is the deceptively consequential logic that assigns each patient to an accountable provider or entity. Methods include **prospective attribution** (assigned in advance, providing population stability and actionability) and **retrospective attribution** (assigned after the fact from where care was actually delivered), using **plurality-of-care** or **primary-care-visit** rules. Misunderstood or inconsistent attribution invalidates every downstream cost and quality comparison; the leader ensures attribution logic is documented, reproducible, and reconciled with the payer's methodology, because the organization is measured against the *payer's* attributed panel, not its own roster.

Quality measure calculation is the other pillar. **Electronic clinical quality measures (eCQMs)** are specified in **CQL (Clinical Quality Language)** with value sets drawn from the **VSAC (Value Set Authority Center)** and structured per the **QDM (Quality Data Model)**; they are reported through programs such as **CMS MIPS**, the **Hospital IQR**, and the **Medicare Shared Savings Program**. The technical demand is precision: a measure has an explicit **initial population, denominator, denominator exclusions/exceptions, and numerator**, and the calculation must match the published specification exactly. Reporting standards have evolved from the legacy **QRDA (Quality Reporting Document Architecture)** toward **FHIR-based quality reporting (the dQM / digital quality measure direction and FHIR Measure/MeasureReport resources)**, consistent with CMS's stated trajectory toward fully digital quality measurement. Senior leaders ensure measure logic is validated against certified results, that the data feeding measures is complete (the data-quality program again proving its worth), and that the organization is not silently failing measures due to mapping or capture gaps rather than true clinical performance.

> **Exam Tip**
> Distinguish *attribution* (which patients count toward whom) from *risk adjustment* (how acuity differences are normalized) from *measure logic* (numerator/denominator definition). Exam scenarios often hinge on one of these three; conflating them is the classic distractor. Also remember eCQMs are specified in CQL with VSAC value sets—not free-form SQL.

.20 Real-World Data, Interoperability-Enabled Analytics, and Privacy

The frontier of health analytics is **real-world data (RWD)**—data generated in routine care (EHRs, claims, registries, devices, patient-generated data)—analyzed to produce **real-world evidence (RWE)** on effectiveness, safety, and outcomes. Scaling RWD analytics depends on interoperability. The **FHIR Bulk Data Access (Flat FHIR)** specification, exposing population data through the **`$export` operation** in newline-delimited JSON, is the standard mechanism for extracting cohort-scale data from EHRs for analytics, quality measurement, and research—operationalized through the **SMART Backend Services** authorization profile for system-to-system, non-interactive access. The **United States Core Data for Interoperability (USCDI)**—a standardized minimum set of data classes and elements expanding annually—defines the common content that certified systems must exchange, giving analytics a predictable, normalized substrate. A senior leader frames Bulk FHIR + USCDI as the path away from brittle, bespoke extracts toward standardized, reusable analytic pipelines.

These capabilities heighten **privacy** obligations. Analytics and secondary use must rest on lawful bases under the **HIPAA Privacy Rule**, and de-identified or limited data should be used wherever the analytic question allows. HIPAA recognizes two **de-identification** routes: **Safe Harbor**, removing 18 specified identifiers (names, dates more specific than year, geographic detail below state with the three-digit ZIP exception, contact and device identifiers, and so on); and **Expert Determination**, in which a qualified statistician certifies that re-identification risk is very small given the data and recipient. Properly de-identified data falls outside HIPAA's restrictions—but the leader must guard against **re-identification** risk from quasi-identifiers and linkage, which intensifies as datasets grow richer.

Between fully identified and de-identified sits the **limited data set (LDS)**: PHI stripped of direct identifiers but retaining certain dates and geographic detail (city, state, ZIP), permissible for research, public health, and operations *only* under a **data use agreement (DUA)** that restricts use and prohibits re-identification. Senior governance must also honor the **minimum necessary** standard for non-de-identified analytics, manage consent and any state-specific or part-2-style sensitive-data constraints, and—when models are trained on patient data—extend privacy review to the model artifacts themselves, since trained models can leak training data. The throughline: interoperability multiplies analytic power and, in equal measure, the leader's accountability for privacy-by-design.

The senior health-IT leader's mandate in analytics is architectural and governing rather than artisanal. The value of any dashboard, model, or population health program is bounded by the platform beneath it—governed data, a single semantic truth, instrumented quality—and by the discipline applied to its lifecycle, from a model's drift-and-bias monitoring to a quality measure's exact specification to a de-identification method's defensibility. Mastery at this level means knowing not merely how to produce an insight, but how to make that insight trustworthy, equitable, reproducible, and safe at enterprise scale.

.21 Chapter 9 Review Questions

Q1. An organization wants a single architecture that stores raw clinical notes, imaging files, and structured EHR extracts in low-cost object storage while still providing ACID transactions, schema enforcement, and high-performance SQL for both BI and machine learning on one copy of the data. Which architecture best meets this requirement?

A) A classic Kimball star-schema enterprise data warehouse only
B) A data lakehouse using an open table format such as Delta Lake or Apache Iceberg
C) A collection of independent departmental data marts with no central store
D) An operational data store fed by real-time HL7 v2 interfaces

Answer: B — The lakehouse pattern, implemented with open table formats (Delta Lake, Iceberg, Hudi), unites schema-on-read lake flexibility for unstructured data with warehouse-grade ACID transactions, schema enforcement, and performance on a single copy—serving BI and ML simultaneously. A classic EDW (A) handles structured data well but is poorly suited to unstructured clinical content; isolated marts (C) and an ODS (D) do not satisfy the unified-storage requirement.

Q2. A care-management program deploys a vendor sepsis-prediction model that validated well at the vendor's reference site. Six months after go-live at the new organization, alert performance has quietly degraded because a new lab analyzer changed the distribution of a key input. Which MLOps concept describes this degradation, and what is the appropriate governance response?

A) Concept drift; retire the model permanently
B) Data drift; the deployed model requires ongoing input-distribution monitoring and re-validation
C) Overfitting; reduce the number of model features
D) Selection bias; exclude the affected patients from analytics

Answer: B — A shift in the input distribution (the new analyzer) is **data drift**. The correct response is continuous monitoring of input/output distributions and a defined re-validation cadence under algorithmic governance—not permanent retirement (A), which is premature. Concept drift (A) refers to a changed input-outcome relationship, overfitting (C) is a training-time problem, and selection bias (D) does not describe this scenario.

Q3. In a Medicare Shared Savings Program ACO, two analysts compute different total-cost-of-care results for "the same" population. Investigation reveals they used different rules for assigning patients to the accountable entity. Which analytic concept is the source of the discrepancy?

A) Risk adjustment
B) Attribution
C) Numerator specification
D) De-identification

Answer: B — **Attribution** logic determines which patients count toward an accountable provider/entity (prospective vs. retrospective, plurality-of-care vs. primary-care-visit rules). Differing attribution rules change the population itself, invalidating downstream cost comparisons. Risk adjustment (A) normalizes acuity but does not select members, numerator specification (C) concerns measure logic, and de-identification (D) is a privacy method.

Q4. An analytics team must extract cohort-scale, population-level data from a certified EHR for quality measurement using a standardized, system-to-system mechanism that returns newline-delimited JSON without interactive user login. Which standard and authorization profile should they use?

A) HL7 v2 ADT feeds with point-to-point VPN
B) FHIR Bulk Data Access (`$export`) with SMART Backend Services authorization
C) A QRDA Category I file emailed nightly
D) Safe Harbor de-identification applied at the interface engine

Answer: B — **FHIR Bulk Data Access (Flat FHIR)** exposes population data via the `$export` operation as newline-delimited JSON, and **SMART Backend Services** provides the non-interactive, system-to-system authorization for it—exactly the standardized cohort-extraction pattern. HL7 v2 ADT (A) is event notification, QRDA (C) is a legacy measure-reporting document not a bulk extraction mechanism, and Safe Harbor (D) is a de-identification method, not a data-access standard.

Q5. A research team requests a dataset that retains admission and discharge dates and patient ZIP codes—data elements removed under HIPAA Safe Harbor—for a treatment-outcomes study. Which mechanism lawfully permits sharing this dataset, and what is required?

A) Fully de-identified data under Safe Harbor; no agreement needed
B) A limited data set under a data use agreement that prohibits re-identification
C) Identified PHI with patient authorization only
D) Expert Determination certifying zero re-identification risk

Answer: B — Because dates and geographic detail (ZIP) are retained, the dataset is not Safe Harbor de-identified; it is a **limited data set (LDS)**, which retains certain dates and geographic detail while removing direct identifiers and may be disclosed for research, public health, or operations **only under a data use agreement (DUA)** that restricts use and prohibits re-identification. Safe Harbor (A) would require removing those very dates and ZIP detail, full authorization (C) is unnecessary for an LDS, and Expert Determination (D) certifies *very small*—not zero—risk and would still require removing or transforming these elements rather than retaining them.

Emerging Technologies, AI Governance, and Innovation Management

Exam Weight: Approximately 10–14 percent (Emerging Technology and Governance)

.22 Learning Objectives

After completing this chapter, the candidate will be able to:

- Design an enterprise innovation pipeline that moves emerging technologies through structured pilots, scaling decisions, and disciplined retirement while accounting for the technology hype cycle.
- Establish an artificial-intelligence governance program for a health system, including an AI governance committee, a model inventory, risk classification, and alignment to the NIST AI Risk Management Framework, the FDA's Software as a Medical Device and Predetermined Change Control Plan pathway, and the EU AI Act high-risk regime.
- Govern the deployment of generative AI and ambient clinical documentation, including bias auditing, ongoing performance monitoring, and human-in-the-loop controls.
- Formulate enterprise cloud strategy—covering multi-cloud, the shared-responsibility model, FinOps, and business associate agreements—and integrate cybersecurity governance using zero-trust principles, the NIST Cybersecurity Framework, third-party risk management, and resilience targets expressed as RTO and RPO.
- Develop interoperability and digital-front-door strategy, including TEFCA and QHIN participation, an API-first FHIR strategy, and an enterprise telehealth model.

.23 Innovation Management and the Enterprise Adoption of Emerging Technology

A senior health-IT leader is not measured by how many emerging technologies the organization touches but by how reliably it converts promising technology into clinical and financial value while avoiding costly distractions. The discipline that governs this conversion is **innovation management**, and at enterprise scale it is operationalized through a formal **innovation pipeline**. The pipeline functions as a funnel: a broad intake of ideas, vendor offerings, and internally generated concepts is progressively filtered through **discovery**, **proof of concept**, **pilot**, **limited production**, and **scale**. Each stage gate has explicit entry and exit criteria, an executive sponsor, a defined budget envelope, and a predetermined kill decision. The single most common failure mode in health systems is the **pilot that never ends**—a perpetual "innovation theater" in which a technology is celebrated in a single department but never scaled, retired, or honestly evaluated. Mature programs therefore make the **scaling decision** an explicit, evidence-based event rather than a default drift.

Leaders should locate every candidate technology on the **hype cycle**, the model that describes how expectations for a new technology rise to a "peak of inflated expectations," collapse into a "trough of disillusionment," and then recover along a "slope of enlightenment" toward a "plateau of productivity." The practical value of the hype-cycle frame is timing. Adopting at the peak invites overpayment, immature tooling, and disillusioned clinicians; waiting for the plateau may forfeit competitive advantage. The senior decision is where on the curve a given technology should be engaged given the organization's **risk appetite**, capital position, and strategic priorities. A leading academic medical center may deliberately operate near the peak for a small portfolio of strategic bets, while a community system rationally waits for the slope of enlightenment when reference customers, integration patterns, and total-cost-of-ownership data are available.

Effective innovation governance separates **sustaining innovation** (incremental improvement of the core EHR and revenue cycle) from **disruptive innovation** (technologies that could reshape the care or business model). The two require different funding, governance, and tolerance for failure. Disruptive bets belong in a portfolio with explicit permission to fail; sustaining work belongs in standard portfolio management. The leader also institutionalizes **technology scouting**, structured vendor evaluation, and partnership models with academic labs and startups, and ties every pipeline stage to a **value realization** measurement plan so that benefits are tracked after go-live, not merely projected before it.

> **Exam Tip**
> When a scenario describes a technology stuck in perpetual pilot, the CPHIMS-aligned answer is to apply a stage-gate scaling decision with defined exit criteria—either scale, sunset, or formally extend with a new success metric. "Continue the pilot indefinitely" and "expand without evaluation" are distractors.

.24 Artificial Intelligence and Generative AI Governance

Artificial intelligence has moved from peripheral analytics to the clinical and operational core of health systems, and governance has had to mature accordingly. The foundational structure is an **AI governance committee** (often styled an AI oversight or responsible-AI council) that is **multidisciplinary by design**: clinical leadership, informatics, data science, privacy and security, legal and compliance, health equity, patient representation, and operations. This committee owns the policy, the intake process for new AI use cases, and the authority to approve, condition, or reject deployment. Crucially, AI governance is positioned as an extension of existing **data and IT governance**, not a parallel silo, so that model decisions inherit the organization's data-stewardship, security, and change-management controls.

The committee's first operational artifact is a comprehensive **model inventory**—a living register of every algorithm in use, whether embedded in the EHR, purchased from a vendor, or built in-house. Many systems are surprised to discover dozens of models already running inside vendor products (sepsis predictors, no-show models, coding suggestions, deterioration indices), most of which arrived without formal review. The inventory captures the model's purpose, training data provenance, intended population, performance metrics, the clinical decision it influences, the human oversight in place, and a maintenance owner. Without an inventory, no meaningful governance is possible because the organization cannot enumerate its own risk surface.

Each inventoried model is assigned a **risk classification** proportional to its potential for patient harm and its degree of autonomy. A low-risk model that ranks administrative work queues is governed far more lightly than a high-risk model that influences a diagnostic or treatment decision. Risk classification drives the depth of validation, the frequency of monitoring, and the level of human oversight required. This proportionality is the central governance principle of the **NIST AI Risk Management Framework (AI RMF)**, the voluntary but widely adopted standard organized around four functions: **Govern** (establish the culture, accountability, and policies), **Map** (contextualize the system and its risks), **Measure** (assess, benchmark, and monitor performance, bias, and robustness), and **Manage** (prioritize and act on risks). The companion **Generative AI Profile** extends the framework to the distinct risks of large language models, such as confabulation, data leakage, and prompt injection. Senior leaders should be able to map their internal program to these four functions because they constitute the de facto language of AI governance in U.S. healthcare.

Regulatory classification runs in parallel with internal risk classification. When an algorithm meets the definition of **Software as a Medical Device (SaMD)**—software intended for a medical purpose without being part of a hardware device—it falls under FDA oversight. The FDA's modern posture recognizes that machine-learning models improve over time, which clashes with the traditional rule that material changes to a cleared device require new submission. The agency's answer is the **Predetermined Change Control Plan (PCCP)**, which allows a manufacturer to specify in advance the modifications a model may undergo (for example, periodic retraining on new data within defined performance bounds) and the methods used to validate those changes, so that anticipated updates can be implemented without a new marketing submission. For the health-IT leader, the practical questions are which of the system's deployed tools are FDA-regulated SaMD, whether the vendor maintains an authorized PCCP, and how the organization will validate model updates locally even when the FDA pathway permits them.

A third lens is international. The **EU AI Act** classifies AI systems by risk tier and places most clinical-decision and safety-critical health AI in the **high-risk** category, triggering obligations around risk management, data governance, technical documentation, logging, human oversight, transparency, and post-market monitoring. Even systems based wholly in the United States increasingly encounter the Act through European patients, partners, vendors, or research collaborations, and many global vendors are engineering to the high-risk bar by default. A CPHIMS-level leader does not need to recite the Act's article numbers but must understand that high-risk classification imposes documentation and human-oversight duties that shape vendor selection and contracting.

> **Key Concept**
> The NIST AI Risk Management Framework is a voluntary, risk-based governance framework built on the Govern–Map–Measure–Manage functions; the FDA's Predetermined Change Control Plan is a regulatory mechanism that lets a SaMD model be updated within pre-authorized bounds; the EU AI Act is binding law that places most clinical AI in a high-risk tier. Do not conflate the voluntary framework, the regulatory pathway, and the statute.

.25 Algorithmic Bias, Validation, and Ongoing Monitoring

A model that performs well in aggregate can still harm specific populations, and the governance program must surface this before and after deployment. **Algorithmic bias auditing** evaluates model performance across demographic and clinical subgroups—race and ethnicity, sex, age, language, payer, and geography—to detect **differential performance** that could widen health disparities. The most-cited cautionary case in the field is a widely used population-health risk model that used historical healthcare spending as a proxy for medical need; because less money had historically been spent on Black patients at equivalent illness levels, the model systematically underestimated their need. The lesson institutionalized in governance is that **proxy targets** and **historically biased training data** can encode inequity even when no protected attribute is used as an input. Bias auditing therefore examines outcomes, not just inputs.

Validation is not a one-time event. Models degrade through **data drift** (the input distribution shifts) and **concept drift** (the relationship between inputs and outcomes shifts), both of which are accelerated in healthcare by changes in coding practice, patient mix, care protocols, and even pandemics. Governance therefore requires **ongoing performance monitoring** with predefined thresholds, automated alerting, scheduled revalidation, and a documented **decommissioning** process for models that can no longer be safely sustained. The organization must also resist **automation bias**—the tendency of clinicians to over-trust algorithmic output—by designing **human-in-the-loop** controls, surfacing model confidence and rationale, and preserving the clinician's authority and accountability over the final decision. The maturity test of an AI program is not whether it can deploy a model but whether it can monitor and retire one.

.26 Ambient Clinical Documentation and LLM Deployment Governance

The most visible generative-AI deployment in 2026 health systems is **ambient clinical documentation**, in which an LLM-based system listens to the clinician–patient encounter and drafts a note for clinician review. The value proposition—reduced documentation burden and clinician burnout, more eye contact with patients—is compelling, but the governance demands are substantial. Because the output is a clinical record that drives care, billing, and legal liability, the governing principle is **draft, not autopilot**: the clinician remains the author and must review and attest to every note. Governance must address **confabulation** (the model inventing details not present in the encounter), the accurate handling of negation and uncertainty, and **omission** of clinically significant statements.

Beyond accuracy, **LLM deployment governance** confronts a cluster of risks unique to generative systems. Patient audio and transcripts are protected health information, so the data-flow architecture, retention, and de-identification practices must be specified and contracted. The vendor's use of customer data for **model training** must be explicitly prohibited or tightly controlled in the agreement. **Prompt injection**, **data leakage**, and **hallucinated citations** are recognized failure modes that demand technical guardrails, output validation, and clear scope limits—an ambient scribe should not be answering arbitrary clinical questions. The program should pilot with measured metrics (note quality, edit rate, clinician satisfaction, time saved, error rate), obtain appropriate patient notification or consent consistent with policy and law, and maintain the audit trail necessary to investigate any documentation error. Generative AI used for patient-facing messaging, prior-authorization drafting, or coding carries analogous governance obligations and belongs in the same model inventory and risk-classification process as predictive models.

.27 Enterprise Cloud Strategy and the Shared-Responsibility Model

Health systems have shifted decisively from "lift and shift" to **cloud-native** strategy, and the senior leader owns the enterprise posture rather than tactical migrations. A foundational competency is the **shared-responsibility model**: the cloud provider is responsible for **security *of* the cloud** (the physical infrastructure, hypervisor, and core services), while the customer is responsible for **security *in* the cloud** (data classification, identity and access management, configuration, encryption, and application security). The most frequent breach cause in cloud environments is not a provider failure but a **customer misconfiguration**—a publicly exposed storage bucket or over-permissioned identity. Leaders must ensure the organization understands precisely where the responsibility boundary falls for each service model, because the boundary shifts between infrastructure-, platform-, and software-as-a-service.

Because cloud providers process and store PHI, each must execute a **business associate agreement (BAA)** under HIPAA before any protected data is placed in their environment. The BAA does not transfer the covered entity's accountability; the health system remains responsible for ensuring the configuration and use of cloud services meet HIPAA's safeguards. Strategy decisions also include **multi-cloud** versus single-cloud postures. Multi-cloud can reduce vendor lock-in, improve resilience, and let teams place workloads on best-fit platforms, but it multiplies operational complexity, skills demands, and security surface; many systems pursue a pragmatic primary-plus-secondary posture rather than true symmetric multi-cloud. Data **sovereignty**, residency, and egress constraints further shape placement decisions.

Cloud's consumption-based economics introduce a new financial-management discipline, **FinOps**, which brings engineering, finance, and business teams together to manage cloud cost with accountability and continuous optimization. Without FinOps, cloud spend balloons through idle resources, over-provisioning, and "bill shock." Mature practice includes **tagging and cost allocation** by service line, **rightsizing**, committed-use and reserved-capacity discounts, and visibility dashboards that make consumption a shared responsibility rather than a surprise on the monthly invoice. The leader treats cloud cost as a governed product metric, not an uncontrollable utility bill.

> **Exam Tip**
>
> In any cloud security scenario, remember that signing a BAA and the existence of the shared-responsibility model do **not** transfer the covered entity's accountability for PHI. The customer always retains responsibility for data, identity, and configuration. Answers implying the cloud vendor is "fully responsible for HIPAA compliance" are incorrect.

.28 Cybersecurity Governance, Zero Trust, and Resilience

Healthcare remains among the most-targeted sectors for cyberattack, and cybersecurity is now an enterprise-risk and board-level concern rather than a technical specialty. The governing reference is the **NIST Cybersecurity Framework (CSF) 2.0**, organized around six functions: **Govern** (newly elevated in 2.0 to emphasize cybersecurity as an enterprise-risk-management responsibility with executive accountability), **Identify**, **Protect**, **Detect**, **Respond**, and **Recover**. The framework gives leadership a common vocabulary to assess current state against a target profile and to communicate posture to the board in business terms.

The dominant architectural strategy is **zero-trust architecture**, captured by the maxim "**never trust, always verify**." Zero trust abandons the obsolete assumption that anything inside the network perimeter is safe; instead it continuously authenticates and authorizes every user, device, and workload, enforces **least-privilege** access, and uses **micro-segmentation** to limit lateral movement so that a single compromised credential cannot traverse the enterprise. Implementing zero trust is a multi-year program touching identity, network, endpoint, and application layers, and the leader frames it as a roadmap, not a product purchase.

A large share of healthcare breaches now originate not with the organization but with its suppliers, making **third-party and vendor risk management** a first-order governance domain. The program inventories vendors with access to data or systems, tiers them by risk, conducts security due diligence and ongoing assessment, requires evidence such as SOC 2 reports, and embeds security obligations and breach-notification terms in contracts. The systemic risk of a single critical vendor outage—demonstrated by major clearinghouse and infrastructure disruptions that cascaded across thousands of providers—has made **concentration risk** and **fourth-party** (the vendor's vendors) exposure explicit board concerns.

Ransomware preparedness sits at the center of resilience planning because a successful attack can halt clinical operations for weeks. The leader ensures **immutable, offline, and tested backups** (defending the "3-2-1" principle and air-gapped copies), network segmentation to contain spread, and—critically—a rehearsed response. **Business continuity and disaster recovery (BC/DR)** planning is operationalized through two metrics every CPHIMS candidate must master. The **recovery time objective (RTO)** is the maximum tolerable duration a system can be unavailable before unacceptable harm occurs; it answers "how fast must we be back?" The **recovery point objective (RPO)** is the maximum tolerable amount of data loss measured in time; it answers "how much data can we afford to lose?" An RPO of one hour requires recovery to a state no older than one hour, which dictates backup or replication frequency, while a four-hour RTO dictates the recovery architecture and staffing. These objectives are set per system based on clinical criticality—the EHR demands aggressive targets, an internal wiki does not—and they must be validated through **tabletop exercises** and full **DR tests**, including practiced **downtime procedures** so clinicians can continue safe care when systems are unavailable. A plan that has never been tested is an assumption, not a capability.

> **Key Concept**
>
> RTO measures *time to restore service*; RPO measures *acceptable data loss*. A short RTO drives recovery architecture and failover capacity; a short RPO drives backup and replication frequency. Confusing the two is a classic exam trap—anchor RTO to "downtime" and RPO to "data loss."

.29 Interoperability Strategy and the Digital Front Door

Interoperability has matured from a compliance obligation into a strategic capability, and the senior leader sets enterprise direction rather than negotiating point-to-point interfaces. The national framework is the **Trusted Exchange Framework and Common Agreement (TEFCA)**, which establishes a "network of networks" for nationwide health-information exchange. Participation flows through a **Qualified Health Information Network (QHIN)**—a designated entity that connects networks to one another under common technical and policy rules. The strategic decision for a health system is which QHIN to join (often through its EHR vendor or a regional HIE), how TEFCA participation complements existing exchange relationships, and how the supported **exchange purposes**—treatment, individual access, and increasingly payment and operations—map to organizational priorities.

Underneath the policy framework, the technical lingua franca is **HL7 FHIR (Fast Healthcare Interoperability Resources)**, a RESTful, resource-based standard now mandated by federal rules for standardized API access to clinical data. U.S. regulation (the ONC/ASTP Cures Act rules and CMS interoperability rules) requires certified EHRs to expose standardized FHIR APIs and obligates many payers to provide **Patient Access**, **Provider Directory**, and **Payer-to-Payer** APIs, with newer rules advancing FHIR-based **prior authorization**. The strategic implication is a deliberate move to an **API-first** posture, in which capabilities are exposed and consumed as governed, reusable APIs rather than brittle batch interfaces. An API-first strategy demands an **API gateway**, developer and partner management, versioning discipline, OAuth 2.0 and SMART-on-FHIR authorization, robust logging, and—because open APIs widen the attack surface—security and consent controls integrated from the start. The leader also navigates the federal **information-blocking** rules, which prohibit practices that unreasonably interfere with the access, exchange, or use of electronic health information, with defined exceptions; non-compliance carries financial and reputational consequences.

The patient-facing expression of this strategy is the **digital front door** and the broader **telehealth** model. The digital front door is the integrated set of digital channels—patient portal and app, online scheduling and registration, virtual visits, secure messaging, remote monitoring, AI-assisted symptom navigation, and digital payment—through which patients access and move through care. Strategically it is a single, governed experience rather than a collection of disconnected point solutions, and its success is measured in access, conversion, leakage prevention, and patient experience. **Telehealth** has settled into a durable, hybrid model in which virtual and in-person care are blended by clinical appropriateness; the leader's concerns are reimbursement policy and its periodic shifts, cross-state **licensure**, **remote patient monitoring** integration into clinical workflow, the **digital divide** and equity of access, and the integration of telehealth data back into the longitudinal record so that virtual encounters are first-class clinical events rather than orphaned silos.

> **Exam Tip**
>
> Distinguish the layers of interoperability strategy: **TEFCA/QHIN** is the national policy framework and trust layer; **FHIR** is the technical API standard; **information blocking** is the regulatory prohibition; the **digital front door** is the patient-experience strategy. A strong answer matches the right layer to the scenario rather than treating "interoperability" as one undifferentiated concept.

.30 Conclusion

The emerging-technology and governance domain asks the senior health-IT leader to hold innovation and discipline in the same hand. The leader must run an innovation pipeline that scales winners and retires the rest, govern AI and generative AI through an inventory, risk classification, and frameworks spanning the NIST AI RMF, FDA PCCP, and EU AI Act, deploy cloud and ambient documentation with eyes open to the shared-responsibility boundary and the limits of automation, build cyber-resilience around zero trust and tested RTO/RPO targets, and set an interoperability and digital-front-door strategy anchored in TEFCA, FHIR, and API-first thinking. Across all of these, the recurring exam theme is **proportional, accountable governance**: matching the depth of oversight to the level of risk, and never allowing a framework, a vendor agreement, or a regulatory pathway to displace the organization's own retained accountability.

.31 Chapter 10 Review Questions

Q1. A health system has deployed an AI-based sepsis prediction model embedded in its EHR and is establishing a formal AI governance program. Which action should be the *first* operational priority for the new AI governance committee?

A) Negotiate a Predetermined Change Control Plan with the FDA
B) Create a comprehensive model inventory of all algorithms in use across the enterprise
C) Adopt the EU AI Act high-risk documentation template
D) Purchase a third-party bias-auditing tool

Answer: B — Governance is impossible without first knowing what exists. A comprehensive model inventory enumerates every algorithm—including those already embedded in vendor products—so the committee can classify risk and apply proportional oversight. The PCCP applies only to FDA-regulated SaMD, EU AI Act documentation is a downstream control, and bias tooling presupposes knowing which models to audit. The inventory is the foundational artifact.

Q2. During a business continuity planning exercise, the EHR is assigned an RTO of two hours and an RPO of fifteen minutes. Which statement correctly interprets these objectives?

A) The system must be restored within fifteen minutes, with up to two hours of data loss tolerated
B) Backups must run every two hours, and the system must be fully restored within fifteen minutes
C) The system must be restored to operation within two hours, and recovery must lose no more than fifteen minutes of data
D) Both values describe the maximum acceptable downtime for the system

Answer: C — RTO is the maximum tolerable time to restore service (two hours), driving recovery architecture and failover capacity. RPO is the maximum tolerable data loss measured in time (fifteen minutes), driving backup or replication frequency. Option C correctly assigns each metric; the others invert or conflate the two concepts.

Q3. A health system is moving major workloads to a public cloud provider and has executed a business associate agreement. Under the shared-responsibility model, which of the following remains the *customer's* responsibility?

A) Physical security of the provider's data centers
B) Security of the underlying hypervisor and core infrastructure services
C) Data classification, identity and access management, and configuration of cloud services
D) Patching of the provider's foundational platform services

Answer: C — The cloud provider is responsible for security *of* the cloud (physical infrastructure, hypervisor, core services), while the customer is responsible for security *in* the cloud—data, identity, and configuration.

Most cloud breaches stem from customer misconfiguration. Neither the BAA nor the shared-responsibility model transfers the covered entity's accountability for PHI.

Q4. A community hospital is evaluating an emerging analytics technology that is currently receiving intense industry attention, premium pricing, and immature integration tooling. Using the technology hype-cycle framework, which strategic posture is most defensible for a risk-averse community system?

A) Adopt immediately at the peak of inflated expectations to gain first-mover advantage
B) Wait for the slope of enlightenment, when reference customers and total-cost-of-ownership data are available
C) Reject the technology permanently to avoid all risk
D) Begin an open-ended pilot with no defined exit criteria

Answer: B — Adopting at the peak invites overpayment, immature tooling, and clinician disillusionment. A risk-averse community system rationally waits for the slope of enlightenment, when reference customers, proven integration patterns, and reliable cost data reduce risk. Permanent rejection forfeits future value, and an open-ended pilot with no exit criteria is the "perpetual pilot" antipattern.

Q5. A health system is deploying an LLM-based ambient clinical documentation tool. Which governance control most directly addresses the risk of the model fabricating clinical details (confabulation) in the generated note?

A) Signing a BAA with the ambient documentation vendor
B) Requiring clinician review and attestation of every generated note before it enters the record
C) Adding the tool to the enterprise model inventory
D) Encrypting the audio transcripts at rest

Answer: B — Confabulation—the model inventing details not present in the encounter—is mitigated by keeping the clinician as the accountable author through mandatory review and attestation ("draft, not autopilot"), with human-in-the-loop oversight. A BAA addresses PHI handling, the inventory enables governance broadly, and encryption protects data at rest; none of these directly catches a fabricated clinical statement before it reaches the record.

IT Financial Management, Vendor and Contract Strategy, and Organizational Leadership

Exam Weight: Approximately 14–18 percent (Administration, Leadership, and Management domain)

.32 Learning Objectives

After completing this chapter, the candidate will be able to:

- Construct and defend an IT business case using total cost of ownership, return on investment, net present value, internal rate of return, and payback period, and explain the strategic implications of the cap-ex to op-ex shift driven by SaaS.
- Lead a structured procurement and vendor selection process spanning RFI, RFP, and RFQ instruments, weighted scoring, contract negotiation, and the full contract lifecycle, including the specialized clauses required for healthcare engagements.
- Govern ongoing vendor relationships through service level agreements, key performance indicators, business associate agreements, source-code escrow, and continuous vendor risk and performance management.
- Design IT organizational structures and staffing models, differentiate the executive technology roles (CIO, CMIO, CNIO, CISO), and apply evidence-based practices for recruiting, retention, performance management, and succession planning.
- Lead enterprise-scale organizational change using established frameworks such as Kotter and ADKAR, communicate effectively with executives and governing boards, and discharge the ethical and regulatory leadership responsibilities expected of a senior health-IT professional.

.33 IT Financial Management in the Healthcare Enterprise

A senior health-IT leader is, before anything else, a steward of constrained capital. Healthcare delivery organizations operate on thin and volatile margins—frequently in the low single digits—so every dollar directed toward technology competes directly with clinical staffing, facilities, and supply chains. Mastery of the financial vocabulary and disciplines that govern these decisions is therefore not a back-office competency but a core leadership requirement.

The foundational distinction is between **capital expenditure (cap-ex)** and **operating expenditure (op-ex)**. Capital spending acquires or builds assets with a useful life beyond a single fiscal year—servers, network infrastructure, a perpetually licensed electronic health record (EHR) installation, a data center build-out. Such outlays are recorded on the balance sheet and recovered over time through **depreciation**, which spreads the asset's cost across its useful life (commonly via the straight-line method, dividing acquisition cost less salvage value by years of service). Operating spending, by contrast, covers the recurring cost of running the enterprise—staff salaries, maintenance contracts, cloud subscriptions, electricity—and is expensed in the period incurred. The two budgets are typically governed by different approval bodies and different fiscal rules: capital budgets are often set annually through a competitive capital allocation committee that ranks projects across the entire organization, while operating budgets are managed at the departmental level against a fixed annual envelope.

The most consequential financial trend of the past decade is the migration from cap-ex to op-ex driven by **Software as a Service (SaaS)** and cloud delivery. A perpetual-license EHR purchased outright is a capital asset depreciated over five to seven years; the same capability consumed as a subscription is a recurring operating expense with no asset on the books. This shift has profound managerial consequences. It lowers the up-front cash barrier and shortens time to value, but it converts a one-time hurdle into a perpetual, often escalating, operating liability that consumes the operating budget indefinitely. Cloud consumption is elastic and metered, which complicates forecasting and can produce "bill shock" without disciplined **FinOps** (cloud financial operations) governance. The senior leader must recognize that a SaaS decision is not merely a sourcing choice but a balance-sheet strategy that affects cash flow, tax treatment, and the predictability of future budgets.

Total cost of ownership (TCO) is the analytic device that prevents the most common procurement error: anchoring on the purchase price. TCO captures the complete lifetime cost of a system—acquisition, implementation and integration, training, interfaces, ongoing licensing and maintenance, infrastructure, internal support staff, downtime, and eventual decommissioning and data migration. In healthcare, the indirect and "soft" costs—physician productivity loss during go-live, clinical workflow redesign, the interface engine work to connect a new ancillary system to the EHR—frequently dwarf the sticker price and are precisely the costs that naïve comparisons omit. A rigorous TCO model spanning the full expected service life is the only honest basis for comparing a SaaS subscription against an on-premises license.

> **Key Concept**
>
> Total cost of ownership is evaluated over the full system lifecycle, not the contract term. A SaaS offering with a low first-year subscription may exceed a perpetual license on a five-year TCO basis once recurring fees, integration, and internal support are fully loaded. Always normalize competing options to the same multi-year horizon before comparing.

.34 Business Cases, Capital Justification, and Investment Analysis

No significant health-IT investment should proceed without a formal **business case**—a structured document that articulates the problem or opportunity, the strategic alignment, the options considered (including the "do nothing" baseline), the costs and benefits of each, the risks, and a clear recommendation. The business case is the leader's instrument for translating technical ambition into financial language the finance committee and board can evaluate. A credible business case quantifies benefits wherever possible (reduced length of stay, decreased denied claims, avoided overtime, FTE redeployment) and is explicit about which benefits are *cashable* (they reduce real spending) versus *non-cashable* (they create capacity or quality improvements that do not directly free cash).

Several quantitative techniques translate cost-benefit estimates into decision metrics. **Return on investment (ROI)** expresses net benefit as a percentage of cost—net benefits divided by total cost—and is intuitive but ignores the timing of cash flows. **Payback period** measures how long until cumulative benefits recover the initial outlay; it is simple and favored for liquidity-sensitive organizations but is blind to anything occurring after the recovery point and to the time value of money.

The more rigorous metrics incorporate the time value of money through **discounting. Net present value (NPV)** discounts all projected cash inflows and outflows back to today's dollars using a **discount rate** (typically the organization's weighted average cost of capital) and sums them; a positive NPV indicates the project creates value, and among competing projects the higher NPV is preferred. **Internal rate of return (IRR)** is the discount rate at which NPV equals zero—conceptually, the project's intrinsic yield—and is compared against the organization's **hurdle rate**, the minimum acceptable return. A project clears the financial bar only if its IRR exceeds the hurdle rate and its NPV is positive. The senior candidate should understand that NPV is generally the superior decision criterion when projects differ in scale or cash-flow timing, because IRR can mislead when comparing mutually exclusive projects of different sizes.

Chargeback and **showback** are the mechanisms by which IT costs are made visible and allocated to the business units that consume them. Under a chargeback model, IT services are billed to consuming departments based on actual or apportioned usage, creating real budget accountability and discouraging waste. Showback presents the same consumption data without actually transferring funds—an informational discipline that builds cost awareness with less political friction. Mature organizations use these models to shift IT from an opaque cost center toward a transparent service provider whose value can be measured. The leader must balance the behavioral benefits of cost transparency against the administrative overhead and the risk that aggressive chargeback drives "shadow IT" as departments route around perceived overcharges.

> **Exam Tip**
>
> Know the distinguishing weakness of each investment metric. ROI ignores timing; payback ignores both the time value of money and post-payback cash flows; NPV and IRR both discount but IRR can produce misleading rankings

for mutually exclusive projects of different scale. When the exam asks which metric to recommend for a long-horizon capital decision, NPV is usually the defensible answer.

.35 Procurement, Vendor Selection, and the Sourcing Process

Healthcare IT is overwhelmingly delivered through vendors, so the discipline of acquiring and governing those relationships is central to senior management. The sourcing process is structured around three instruments that are frequently confused and routinely tested. A **Request for Information (RFI)** is an early, low-commitment instrument used to survey the market, understand available capabilities, and shape requirements before any intent to buy is signaled; it gathers intelligence, not bids. A **Request for Proposal (RFP)** is issued when requirements are defined but the optimal solution is not, inviting vendors to propose how they would meet stated needs and to be evaluated on capability, approach, references, and price together; the RFP is the workhorse of complex healthcare procurements such as EHR or enterprise imaging selection. A **Request for Quote (RFQ)** is appropriate when the requirement is precisely specified and commoditized, so that price is the principal differentiator—hardware refreshes, additional licenses of an already-selected product.

Vendor selection should be governed by a documented, **weighted scoring** methodology agreed upon *before* proposals are opened, to insulate the decision from bias and from a single charismatic demonstration. Evaluation criteria typically span functional fit, technical architecture and interoperability, security and compliance posture, total cost of ownership, vendor viability and financial stability, implementation methodology, reference quality, and cultural fit. Each criterion carries a predetermined weight reflecting strategic priority; each vendor is scored against each criterion, often by a cross-functional committee including clinicians, IT, security, finance, supply chain, and legal; and the weighted scores are summed. Structured scripted demonstrations, site visits to live reference clients, and direct reference checks (including references the vendor did *not* supply) are essential validation steps. A senior leader manages the selection process to be defensible, transparent, and resistant to the "champion" dynamic in which an internal sponsor's enthusiasm overrides objective evaluation.

.36 Contracts, Service Levels, and the Specialized Clauses of Healthcare IT

Selection culminates in a contract, and the **contract lifecycle**—negotiation, execution, ongoing administration, performance monitoring, amendment, renewal, and termination—is a continuous management responsibility, not a one-time legal event. Several contractual structures deserve senior-level command.

Service level agreements (SLAs) define the measurable performance the vendor commits to deliver—uptime (often expressed as a percentage such as 99.9 percent, with the leader translating that into permissible annual downtime), response and resolution times for incidents by severity, and support availability. SLAs must specify the **key performance indicators (KPIs)** that operationalize them, the measurement method, the reporting cadence, and—critically—the **service credits** or remedies that apply when targets are missed. A common and costly oversight is an SLA with metrics but no meaningful financial consequence for breach; without remedies, an SLA is merely an aspiration.

Software licensing models vary widely and carry materially different cost and compliance profiles: perpetual licenses with annual maintenance, term or subscription licenses, named-user versus concurrent-user models, capacity- or transaction-based metering, and modern consumption-based cloud pricing. Each demands a different forecasting and license-management discipline; under-licensing exposes the organization to true-up penalties on audit, while over-licensing wastes capital.

Two clauses are nearly unique to mission-critical and healthcare contexts. **Source-code escrow** protects the organization against vendor failure: the vendor deposits source code with a neutral third party, to be released to the customer under defined trigger conditions (bankruptcy, abandonment, breach), preserving the ability to maintain a critical system if the vendor disappears. The **Business Associate Agreement (BAA)** is a HIPAA-mandated contract required of any vendor that creates, receives, maintains, or transmits protected health information on the covered entity's behalf; it obligates the business associate to safeguard PHI, restrict use and disclosure, report breaches, and flow equivalent obligations to its own subcontractors. The senior leader must ensure that no vendor touches PHI without an executed BAA and that the BAA is refreshed as services and subcontractor chains evolve. Additional protective clauses to negotiate include data ownership and portability (the right to extract your data in a usable format at termination), price-escalation caps, audit rights, indemnification, limitation-of-liability terms calibrated to the risk, and a defined exit and transition-services plan.

> **Key Concept**
> A Business Associate Agreement is a legal prerequisite, not a courtesy. Under HIPAA, a covered entity may not permit a vendor to handle protected health information without an executed BAA, and the covered entity retains compliance accountability for its business associates. Verify BAA coverage for every vendor in the PHI chain, including downstream subcontractors and cloud hosting providers.

.37 Vendor Relationship, Risk, and Performance Management

The contract signing marks the beginning, not the end, of vendor management. **Vendor performance management** is the ongoing discipline of holding vendors to their SLAs and KPIs through regular operational reviews, scorecards, and escalation when performance drifts. Effective programs segment vendors by strategic importance—a small number of strategic partners whose systems are mission-critical warrant deep, executive-level relationship management, while transactional commodity suppliers are managed with lighter governance. This tiering focuses scarce relationship-management energy where business risk is concentrated.

Vendor risk management has expanded dramatically as the healthcare attack surface has shifted toward the supply chain. Third-party and fourth-party (your vendor's vendors) risk now drives a large share of healthcare data breaches, and regulators and boards expect a formal **third-party risk management (TPRM)** program. Such a program assesses each vendor's security posture before onboarding (security questionnaires, evidence of SOC 2 Type II reports or HITRUST certification, penetration-test summaries), establishes contractual security and breach-notification obligations, and re-assesses periodically across the relationship's life. The leader must maintain an accurate inventory of all vendors with access to systems or data, classify them by the sensitivity of that access, and ensure continuous rather than point-in-time assurance.

Post-implementation relationship management also encompasses managing the inevitable tension between partner and supplier. The leader cultivates a relationship constructive enough to gain influence over the product roadmap and responsive support, while preserving the leverage—renewal timing, reference value, competitive alternatives, contractual remedies—needed to enforce commitments. Joint governance forums, executive sponsor pairings, and a documented issue-escalation path keep the relationship healthy and prevent small service failures from metastasizing into adversarial disputes.

.38 Negotiation Fundamentals for the Senior Leader

Negotiation competence underlies both procurement and ongoing vendor management. The senior leader should approach negotiation as a search for value rather than a zero-sum contest, distinguishing **positions** (what each side says it wants) from **interests** (the underlying needs that explain those positions). The strongest source of leverage is the **BATNA**—the Best Alternative To a Negotiated Agreement—because a credible, prepared alternative (a runner-up vendor, an internal build option, a willingness to extend the status quo) defines the point below which no deal is acceptable. Establishing and protecting a strong BATNA, and understanding the counterparty's BATNA, is the foundation of negotiating power.

Practical levers in software negotiation include the timing of the deal (vendors discount heavily at quarter- and year-end to make their numbers), bundling and volume, multi-year commitments traded for price-escalation caps, and the deliberate sequencing of which terms are conceded. The leader should negotiate the *entire* lifetime relationship—renewal pricing, support escalation, professional-services rates, and exit terms—at the moment of greatest leverage, which is *before* signing, because leverage collapses once the organization is dependent on a deployed system (the "lock-in" problem). Negotiating a favorable initial price while ceding uncapped future escalation is a classic and expensive trap.

.39 Human-Capital Leadership and IT Organizational Design

Technology delivers value only through people, and the senior health-IT leader's most durable contribution is the organization and the talent they build. **IT organizational structures** range from centralized models (a single enterprise IT function with consistent standards and economies of scale) through decentralized models (IT embedded in business units for responsiveness) to **federated or hybrid** models that centralize infrastructure, security, and standards while distributing analysts and application support to clinical and operational areas. There is no universally correct structure; the leader selects and evolves the model to match the organization's size, geographic dispersion, and strategic priorities, recognizing the perpetual trade-off between standardization and local responsiveness.

The executive technology roles must be clearly differentiated, a frequent exam topic. The **Chief Information Officer (CIO)** owns the overall information-systems strategy, infrastructure, budget, and IT operations, and sits as the senior technology voice in the executive suite. The **Chief Medical Information Officer (CMIO)**—typically a practicing physician—bridges clinical practice and IT, owning physician adoption, clinical decision support, and the alignment of systems with medical workflow. The **Chief Nursing Informatics Officer (CNIO)** performs the analogous role for nursing, the largest clinical workforce and the heaviest EHR users, championing nursing workflow and documentation efficiency. The **Chief Information Security Officer (CISO)** owns the security and risk program, increasingly reporting independently (to the CEO, board, or chief risk officer rather than solely to the CIO) to preserve the objectivity needed to challenge IT decisions on security grounds. A growing number of organizations also designate a **Chief Health Information Officer (CHIO)** or a **Chief Digital Officer** to lead digital-health and patient-experience transformation. Clarity about these roles' distinct accountabilities prevents the gaps and overlaps that undermine governance.

Staffing models must balance internal employees, contractors, and managed-service or outsourced arrangements, calibrated to the difference between durable core competencies (which belong in-house) and surge or specialized needs (which may be sourced externally). The leader faces an acute and persistent **recruiting and retention** challenge: health-IT skills—particularly in security, data engineering, integration, and cloud—are scarce and mobile, and competition extends well beyond healthcare to higher-paying technology employers. Evidence-based retention practices emphasize meaningful work and mission, clear career-development pathways, competitive and equitable compensation, flexible and remote work options, recognition, and—above all—the quality of frontline management, since people leave managers more often than they leave organizations.

Performance management at the senior level means setting clear, measurable objectives aligned to organizational strategy, providing continuous feedback rather than relying solely on annual reviews, and differentiating performance so that high performers are recognized and developed while underperformance is addressed candidly and promptly. Building **high-performing teams** requires psychological safety (the shared belief that members can take interpersonal risks without humiliation), clarity of roles and goals, and a culture of accountability—qualities the leader must deliberately cultivate rather than assume. Finally, **succession planning** safeguards organizational continuity: the leader identifies critical roles, assesses bench strength, develops internal candidates through stretch assignments and mentoring, and documents knowledge to mitigate the operational risk concentrated in a few irreplaceable individuals. A leader who has built no successor has, by definition, not finished the job.

.40 Change Leadership and Organizational Change Management at Scale

Enterprise health-IT initiatives fail far more often from organizational resistance than from technical defect. **Organizational change management (OCM)** is therefore an indispensable leadership discipline, distinct from project management: where project management governs scope, schedule, and budget, OCM governs the human transition that determines whether the technical deliverable is actually adopted and sustained.

Two frameworks dominate professional practice and the exam. **Kotter's eight-step model** approaches change at the organizational level: establish a sense of urgency; build a guiding coalition; form a strategic vision and initiatives; enlist a volunteer army; enable action by removing barriers; generate short-term wins; sustain acceleration; and institute change in the culture. Kotter's emphasis on urgency, coalition, and embedding change durably in culture makes it well suited to large-scale transformations such as an enterprise EHR transition. The **ADKAR model** complements Kotter by working at the level of the individual, recognizing that organizations change only when their people do. ADKAR specifies five sequential outcomes each affected person must achieve: **A**wareness of the need for change, **D**esire to participate and support it, **K**nowledge of how to change, **A**bility to implement the required skills and behaviors, and **R**einforcement to sustain the change. Its power lies in diagnosis: when adoption stalls, the leader can identify which barrier point (awareness, desire, knowledge, ability, or reinforcement) is blocking a specific group and target the intervention accordingly. The sophisticated leader uses Kotter to orchestrate the enterprise campaign and ADKAR to manage the individual transitions within it, supported by stakeholder analysis, a communication plan, super-user networks, and reinforcement mechanisms that prevent regression after go-live.

> **Exam Tip**
> Map the two change frameworks to their level of action. Kotter's eight steps operate at the *organizational* level and stress urgency, a guiding coalition, and anchoring change in culture. ADKAR operates at the *individual* level—Awareness, Desire, Knowledge, Ability, Reinforcement—and is the better diagnostic for pinpointing why a specific group is resisting adoption.

.41 Stakeholder Communication, Ethics, and Regulatory Leadership

Senior leaders are judged substantially on their ability to communicate up and out. Communicating with **executives and governing boards** requires translating technical complexity into the language of risk, value, and strategy—concise, decision-oriented, and free of jargon. Boards increasingly expect routine reporting on cybersecurity posture, major-project status, and technology risk, and the leader who can frame a security investment as enterprise risk mitigation, or an EHR optimization as a quality and financial return, earns the credibility and capital that technical fluency alone never will. **Stakeholder management** more broadly means systematically identifying the parties affected by an initiative, analyzing their influence and interest, and tailoring engagement so that powerful and interested stakeholders are managed closely while others are kept appropriately informed.

Professional ethics anchors all of this. HIMSS maintains a **Code of Ethics** for health information and technology professionals built on principles of integrity, accountability, confidentiality and privacy, and acting in the patient's and public's best interest. Senior leaders confront ethical questions that are rarely black-and-white—the secondary use of patient data, conflicts of interest in vendor selection, the equitable allocation of scarce IT resources, transparency about system limitations, and the responsible governance of artificial intelligence in clinical settings, where questions of bias, transparency, and accountability are now front and center. The ethical leader models candor, declares and recuses from conflicts of interest, protects the confidentiality of patient and proprietary information, and ensures that decisions can withstand public scrutiny.

Finally, **regulatory and compliance leadership** is a non-delegable senior responsibility. The leader ensures organizational adherence to HIPAA's Privacy and Security Rules, the Breach Notification Rule, the information-blocking provisions and interoperability requirements advanced under the 21st Century Cures Act and enforced by the Office of the National Coordinator, and the evolving landscape of state privacy laws and federal cybersecurity expectations. This means not merely achieving point-in-time compliance but building a sustainable compliance program—policies, training, monitoring, auditing, and a documented response capability—and fostering a culture in which compliance is understood as integral to patient trust rather than as bureaucratic friction. The senior health-IT leader who integrates financial discipline, vendor governance, human-capital development, change leadership, and ethical regulatory stewardship into a coherent practice embodies the management competencies the CPHIMS credential is designed to certify.

.42 Chapter 11 Review Questions

Q1. A health system is comparing a perpetually licensed on-premises EHR against a SaaS subscription EHR. To make a financially honest comparison, the CIO insists the analysis capture acquisition, implementation, integration, training, ongoing licensing, internal support staff, and decommissioning costs across a five-year horizon. Which financial concept is the CIO applying?

A) Return on investment
B) Total cost of ownership
C) Internal rate of return
D) Chargeback allocation

Answer: B — Total cost of ownership captures the complete lifetime cost of a system across acquisition, implementation, integration, training, ongoing operating costs, internal support, and decommissioning, evaluated over the full service life. ROI, IRR, and chargeback are distinct concepts; only TCO describes the comprehensive lifetime-cost comparison being performed.

Q2. A capital committee must choose between two mutually exclusive IT projects of very different scale and cash-flow timing. The committee wants the single most defensible metric for selecting the option that creates the most value for the organization. Which metric should be the primary basis for the decision?

A) Payback period, because it measures liquidity recovery
B) Return on investment, because it is the simplest percentage
C) Net present value, because it discounts all cash flows and is reliable across differing project scales
D) Internal rate of return, because the higher percentage always indicates the better project

Answer: C — Net present value discounts all projected cash flows to present dollars and, unlike IRR, ranks mutually exclusive projects of different scale reliably. Payback ignores the time value of money and post-payback flows; ROI ignores timing; IRR can mislead when comparing projects of differing size. NPV is the defensible choice for a long-horizon, mutually-exclusive capital decision.

Q3. An organization needs to acquire a complex enterprise imaging solution. The requirements are well understood, but the best technical approach and vendor are not yet determined, and the organization wants vendors to propose how they would meet the needs and be evaluated on capability, references, and price together. Which procurement instrument is most appropriate?

A) Request for Information (RFI)
B) Request for Quote (RFQ)
C) Request for Proposal (RFP)
D) Business Associate Agreement (BAA)

Answer: C — An RFP is used when requirements are defined but the optimal solution is not, inviting vendors to propose approaches evaluated on capability, references, and price together. An RFI gathers early market intelligence with no intent to buy; an RFQ is for precisely specified, commoditized purchases where price dominates; a BAA is a HIPAA contract, not a sourcing instrument.

Q4. During an enterprise EHR rollout, clinician adoption has stalled in one department. Leadership determines that the clinicians understand why the change is happening and are willing to participate, but they have not yet acquired the specific skills to use the new documentation workflow effectively. Using the ADKAR model, which element is the current barrier?

A) Awareness
B) Desire
C) Ability
D) Reinforcement

Answer: C — In ADKAR (Awareness, Desire, Knowledge, Ability, Reinforcement), the clinicians already have awareness and desire; the barrier is Ability—the capacity to implement the required skills and behaviors in practice. The targeted intervention is hands-on training and at-the-elbow support to build that ability, not further messaging about the need for change.

Q5. A cloud vendor will host an application that stores and transmits protected health information on behalf of a covered entity. Before the vendor is permitted to handle the PHI, which contractual instrument is a legal prerequisite under HIPAA, and what additional protection should the leader negotiate to guard against the vendor's potential business failure?

A) A service level agreement; and a price-escalation cap
B) A Business Associate Agreement; and source-code escrow
C) A Request for Proposal; and a chargeback model
D) A statement of work; and a showback report

Answer: B — HIPAA requires an executed Business Associate Agreement before any vendor creates, receives, maintains, or transmits PHI on the covered entity's behalf, obligating the vendor to safeguard PHI and flow obligations to subcontractors. Source-code escrow protects continuity of a critical system if the vendor fails by releasing deposited code under defined trigger conditions. The other options are either not legal prerequisites or address unrelated concerns.

.43 Practice Examination Two

This is the second of two 50-item practice examinations approximating the content proportions of the CPHIMS examination across its three weighted domains—General (the healthcare environment, technology, and regulatory context), Systems (analysis, design, selection, implementation, testing, support, and maintenance), and Administration (leadership, management, and privacy/security). Questions Q1 through Q25 constitute the first half of this form. Allow approximately 1.5 minutes per item, or about 75 minutes for the full 50-question form, which mirrors the pacing of the live computer-based examination. Read each scenario stem carefully, eliminate clearly incorrect options, and select the single best answer; many items are written at a director or manager level and reward recognizing the correct framework, standard, or governing principle rather than recalling a definition in isolation. Rationales follow each item so you can review your reasoning immediately or defer review until you complete the set.

Q1. A newly appointed director of clinical informatics inherits an application portfolio that has grown through acquisition and one-off purchases, with redundant systems and no documented relationship between technology investments and clinical strategy. The CIO asks the director to establish a repeatable, vendor-neutral method for aligning the portfolio with the health system's long-term clinical and financial goals. The director wants a framework that explicitly separates business architecture, data architecture, application architecture, and technology architecture, and that provides an iterative development method for moving from a documented baseline state to an agreed target state with transition steps in between. Which framework most directly meets this need?

A) ITIL 4 Service Value System
B) COBIT 2019 governance objectives
C) The Open Group Architecture Framework (TOGAF) Architecture Development Method
D) PMBOK process groups

Answer: C — TOGAF's Architecture Development Method (ADM) is purpose-built for enterprise architecture and explicitly organizes work into the four architecture domains—business, data, application, and technology—while providing an iterative phased cycle (Preliminary, then Phases A through H, plus Requirements Management at the center) for transitioning from a documented baseline to an agreed target state. The ADM also produces an Architecture Vision and a set of transition architectures, which is precisely what a director needs to rationalize a redundant, acquisition-grown portfolio and sequence change against strategy. ITIL governs IT service management (how services are designed, delivered, and supported), COBIT governs enterprise IT governance (how the board ensures value and manages risk), and the PMBOK Guide governs project delivery (how a single endeavor is planned and executed). None of those three defines the four architecture domains or supplies an architecture transition method, so each is a distractor that names a real framework operating at the wrong layer of abstraction for an enterprise-architecture problem.

Q2. During the organization's annual HIPAA Security Rule risk analysis, a security manager identifies that an unencrypted backup tape containing 40,000 patient records is stored in an unlocked supply closet at a branch clinic accessible to non-clinical staff and contractors. The manager must characterize this finding for the enterprise risk register so leadership can prioritize remediation against other findings. Working from the standard NIST-based risk-analysis model that OCR references, which two elements combine to determine the *level of risk* for this finding?

A) Cost of remediation and budget availability
B) Likelihood that a threat will exploit a vulnerability and the impact (magnitude of harm) if it does
C) Number of records and the encryption algorithm strength
D) Regulatory penalty schedule and the organization's prior breach history

Answer: B — The NIST SP 800-30 risk-analysis methodology that OCR references for HIPAA Security Rule compliance defines the level of risk as a function of the *likelihood* that a particular threat-source will successfully exploit a particular vulnerability and the *impact*, or magnitude of harm, that would result. An unencrypted, physically unsecured tape combines a high likelihood of unauthorized access with a high impact (40,000 records), producing a high risk rating that drives prioritized remediation such as encryption and physical access controls. Note that record count and penalty exposure feel relevant because they influence impact, but on their own they do not constitute the risk equation—likelihood must also be assessed. Remediation cost, encryption strength, and prior-breach history are inputs that inform risk treatment and prioritization decisions rather than the two factors that define the risk level itself, which is why each alternative is incorrect.

Q3. A health system is selecting a new enterprise scheduling system to replace three departmental tools. The selection committee includes representatives from clinical operations, finance, IT, and compliance, and members disagree about how much weight to give upfront license price versus long-term value. The director chairing the committee wants a structured, repeatable way to compare three finalist vendors against criteria such as interoperability, total cost of ownership, usability, and vendor viability, and to be able to defend the outcome if a losing vendor protests. Which selection technique best supports a defensible, transparent comparison?

A) Lowest-bid award to the cheapest license cost
B) A weighted scoring matrix applied to a standardized RFP response
C) Sole-source negotiation with the incumbent vendor
D) A reverse auction limited to upfront price

Answer: B — A weighted scoring matrix applied to standardized RFP responses lets the committee assign relative importance (weights) to each criterion, score each vendor against the same rubric, and compute a defensible composite score, producing a transparent and auditable selection decision that survives later challenge. This method also forces the divided committee to make its priorities explicit—agreeing, for example, that interoperability and total cost of ownership outweigh upfront license price—before any vendor scores are tallied, which reduces the influence of individual bias and gives a losing vendor a documented, objective record if it protests. Lowest-bid award, sole-source negotiation, and reverse auctions each optimize a single dimension (price or incumbency) and ignore the multi-criteria trade-offs that drive long-term value. They are poor fits for a strategic enterprise system selection where usability, vendor viability, and interoperability materially affect outcomes, so each alternative sacrifices the defensibility and balance the director is seeking. The weighted scoring matrix is therefore the only listed technique that satisfies both the committee's need for transparency and its need to account for long-term value beyond upfront price.

Q4. A hospital's interface team must establish a real-time feed of admit, discharge, and transfer (ADT) events between its legacy registration system and its laboratory information system so that the lab always has current patient location and encounter data. Both systems are mature, are connected through the organization's interface engine, and already speak a widely adopted, message-based clinical standard. The IT manager wants to use the established standard rather than build a custom API, minimizing integration risk and ongoing maintenance. Which standard is most appropriate for this real-time, event-driven ADT messaging?

A) DICOM
B) NCPDP SCRIPT
C) HL7 Version 2.x messaging
D) X12 837

Answer: C — HL7 Version 2.x remains the dominant standard for real-time, event-driven clinical messaging within and between hospital systems, and ADT trigger events (A01 admit, A03 discharge, A08 update, and so on) are core to its event taxonomy, carried in pipe-and-hat delimited segments such as MSH, PID, and PV1. Because both the registration and laboratory systems are mature and already speak this message-based standard through the interface engine, an HL7 V2.x interface is the lowest-risk, best-fit choice for the intramural ADT feed and avoids the cost and risk of a custom API. DICOM handles medical imaging objects and metadata, NCPDP SCRIPT handles e-prescribing transactions between prescribers and pharmacies, and X12 837 handles administrative claims submission to payers. None of those three is designed for event-driven ADT messaging between clinical systems, so each is a domain-mismatched distractor even though all are legitimate healthcare standards.

Q5. A manager proposes acquiring a third-party clinical decision support module whose license is modestly priced but which will require interface development, clinician training, content subscriptions, and ongoing maintenance. The CIO is skeptical that the headline license cost reflects the true commitment and asks the manager to justify the investment using a metric that captures the full lifecycle cost—acquisition, implementation, training, maintenance, support, and eventual retirement—rather than just the purchase price. Which financial concept is the CIO requesting?

A) Net present value (NPV)
B) Total cost of ownership (TCO)
C) Internal rate of return (IRR)
D) Payback period

Answer: B — Total cost of ownership (TCO) explicitly aggregates all direct and indirect costs across an asset's full lifecycle—acquisition, implementation, training, interfaces, ongoing maintenance, support, and eventual decommissioning—so leadership can compare alternatives on the basis of what each will truly cost over time rather than sticker price. In health IT, where licensing is often a small fraction of multi-year operating cost, TCO frequently reverses a decision that upfront price alone would have made—a cheap license with expensive interfaces and content subscriptions can cost more over five years than a higher-priced turnkey product. NPV and IRR are discounted-return metrics and payback period measures how quickly an investment recovers its cost; all three consume cost inputs but none of them enumerates lifecycle costs. They answer "is it worth it?" or "how fast do we recoup?" rather than the "what will it truly cost to own?" question the CIO is posing, which is exactly what TCO is built to answer.

Q6. A regional health information exchange (HIE) currently connects hospitals and practices within one state through point-to-point and hub agreements. Its board wants to participate in nationwide data sharing without negotiating a separate legal contract with every external network it might connect to. The HIE's leadership is evaluating the federal framework that was established to create a "network of networks," providing a single common agreement and a shared technical floor for interoperability across the United States. Which initiative is this?

A) Meaningful Use Stage 3
B) The Trusted Exchange Framework and Common Agreement (TEFCA)
C) The Promoting Interoperability Program
D) The 21st Century Cures Act information-blocking penalties

Answer: B — The Trusted Exchange Framework and Common Agreement (TEFCA), mandated by the 21st Century Cures Act and operationalized by ASTP/ONC through the Recognized Coordinating Entity (The Sequoia Project), establishes a common legal agreement and a technical floor so that Qualified Health Information Networks can exchange data nationwide as a "network of networks." For a regional HIE, participating typically means connecting through or becoming part of a QHIN and adopting the Common Agreement's terms and FHIR-based exchange roadmap, which eliminates the need to negotiate a separate legal agreement with every counterparty. Meaningful Use and the Promoting Interoperability programs are CMS incentive and reporting programs tied to certified EHR use, not exchange frameworks, and the information-blocking provisions are a regulatory prohibition that constrains behavior rather than a structure enabling connection. Because only TEFCA establishes a single common agreement plus a technical floor for nationwide "network of networks" exchange, the other options are distractors that name real but different federal initiatives.

Q7. A project manager is overseeing the implementation of a new pharmacy information system that is on schedule and within budget. Midway through the build, the clinical sponsor requests additional barcode-scanning workflows for medication administration that were not in the original project charter, arguing they are important for patient safety. The project manager recognizes the request may have merit but is concerned about schedule, cost, and downstream testing impacts. To control disruption while still allowing legitimate adjustments to be evaluated and approved, the project manager should route this request through which process?

A) Immediate implementation to satisfy the sponsor
B) An integrated change control process that evaluates scope, schedule, cost, and risk impacts before approval
C) Deferral of all changes until after go-live regardless of merit
D) Escalation directly to the vendor for a quote

Answer: B — Integrated change control evaluates each requested change for its impact across scope, schedule, cost, quality, and risk, documents the analysis, and submits it to a change control board for a formal approve, defer, or reject decision, preventing uncontrolled scope creep while still accommodating genuinely valuable changes such as barcode-scanning safety workflows. The approved change is then reflected in updated scope, schedule, and cost baselines so the plan of record stays accurate and the safety-relevant barcode workflow is implemented in a controlled way. Implementing immediately to please the sponsor invites scope creep and unmanaged risk to a project that is currently on track, blanket deferral of all changes regardless of merit ignores legitimate clinical-safety needs, and routing straight to the vendor for a quote bypasses governance and the impact analysis entirely. Each alternative therefore undermines disciplined project control, which is precisely what integrated change control exists to preserve. By contrast, routing the request through change control lets the safety value of barcode scanning be weighed transparently against the cost and schedule of adding it, so a legitimately important change can still be approved without destabilizing an otherwise healthy project.

Q8. A health system is finalizing a software-as-a-service (SaaS) contract for a cloud-hosted patient portal. Legal and IT are reviewing the agreement package, which already includes a master services agreement and a performance schedule. Because the vendor will create, receive, maintain, and transmit protected health information on the health system's behalf, the compliance officer flags that HIPAA requires a specific additional contractual instrument to be executed before any PHI is shared with the vendor. Which document is mandatory?

A) A service-level agreement (SLA) only
B) A business associate agreement (BAA)
C) A non-disclosure agreement (NDA) only
D) A memorandum of understanding (MOU)

Answer: B — Under the HIPAA Privacy and Security Rules, a covered entity must execute a business associate agreement (BAA) with any vendor that creates, receives, maintains, or transmits PHI on its behalf before sharing that PHI; the BAA contractually binds the business associate to safeguard PHI, restrict its use, report security incidents and breaches, and flow obligations down to subcontractors. A cloud-hosted SaaS patient-portal vendor clearly meets the business-associate definition, so the BAA is mandatory before PHI flows regardless of the master services agreement or performance schedule already in the package. An SLA governs performance levels, an NDA governs confidentiality generally, and an MOU is typically a non-binding understanding; none of these satisfies HIPAA's specific BAA requirement, even though an organization commonly executes an SLA alongside the BAA. The compliance officer is therefore correct that the BAA is the distinct, legally required instrument the package still needs.

Q9. A health system's board has asked the CIO to demonstrate that information technology is being governed, not merely operated. The CIO convenes an IT governance committee and wants to adopt a recognized framework that ensures IT delivers value, optimizes risk, and aligns with enterprise objectives, while drawing a clear line between *governance*—the board-level activities of evaluating options, directing strategy, and monitoring performance—and *management*, the activities of planning, building, running, and monitoring operations. Which framework formalizes this governance-versus-management distinction?

A) HL7 FHIR
B) Lean Six Sigma
C) Agile Scrum
D) COBIT 2019

Answer: D — COBIT 2019 explicitly separates governance objectives—the EDM domain (Evaluate, Direct, Monitor) owned by the board and executive leadership—from management objectives in the APO, BAI, DSS, and MEA domains owned by operational IT, giving the organization a structured way to ensure IT delivers value, optimizes risk, and aligns to enterprise goals. This governance-versus-management split is exactly what the board is seeking when it asks the CIO to demonstrate that IT is governed, not merely operated, and COBIT's design factors and goals cascade help tailor the framework to the organization. FHIR is a data-interoperability standard, Lean Six Sigma is a process-improvement methodology aimed at reducing defects and waste, and Agile Scrum is a software-delivery framework for iterative development. None of those three is an enterprise IT governance framework or formalizes the EDM-versus-management distinction, so each is a distractor that operates at a different layer than board-level IT governance.

Q10. A clinical informatics analyst is preparing the organization's certified EHR for participation in an API-based exchange program. She is mapping the data elements that federal interoperability rules require certified health IT to be able to exchange as a baseline set of standardized clinical data classes—including clinical notes, medications, problems, allergies, and laboratory results—so that any conformant partner can consume them. She needs to cite the standard that defines this minimum, versioned baseline content set. Which standard defines this minimum baseline?

A) ICD-10-CM
B) SNOMED CT
C) LOINC
D) USCDI (United States Core Data for Interoperability)

Answer: D — The United States Core Data for Interoperability (USCDI) defines the standardized set of health data classes (such as Clinical Notes, Medications, Problems, Laboratory, and Patient Demographics) and their constituent data elements that ONC-certified health IT must support for interoperable exchange, and it is updated on a versioned, predictable cadence. It is the baseline content standard the analyst is mapping to, and its versioned expansion over time is how new data classes (such as additional social-determinants or clinical-note elements) become part of required interoperable exchange. ICD-10-CM, SNOMED CT, and LOINC are individual code systems and terminologies that *populate* specific USCDI elements—diagnoses and procedures, clinical findings and problems, and laboratory observations respectively—but none of them, by itself, defines the minimum interoperable exchange data set. They are the vocabularies that give USCDI elements coded meaning, making them components of the answer rather than the baseline the question asks for.

Q11. A director of IT operations must design the support model for a newly implemented EHR that will serve 4,000 end users across inpatient and ambulatory settings. To control cost while preserving response quality, she structures support so that Tier 1 handles password resets and basic how-to questions, Tier 2 handles application configuration and workflow issues requiring analyst expertise, and Tier 3 handles defects that must be escalated to the vendor. This deliberate layering, with escalation from one level to the next as needed, is an example of which service management practice?

A) A tiered service desk / incident escalation model
B) A change advisory board
C) A configuration management database
D) A problem management Pareto analysis

Answer: A — A tiered service desk arranges support into escalating levels of expertise—Tier 1 front-line for routine requests, Tier 2 specialists for configuration and workflow issues, and Tier 3 for vendor or engineering escalation of defects—so that incidents are resolved at the lowest competent level and escalated only when necessary, which is the classic ITIL incident-management and escalation pattern. This structure controls cost by resolving routine issues cheaply at Tier 1, preserves scarce analyst and vendor capacity for genuinely complex problems, and improves first-contact resolution rates. A change advisory board governs the review and approval of changes, a configuration management database (CMDB) stores configuration items and their relationships, and Pareto analysis is a technique for prioritizing problems by frequency or impact. None of those describes the front-line-to-specialist-to-vendor support-tier structure the director designed, so each is an ITIL-adjacent distractor that names a different practice.

Q12. A hospital is modernizing its interoperability strategy to support a marketplace of third-party clinical applications. The enterprise architect wants to expose discrete clinical resources—such as Patient, Observation, and MedicationRequest—over RESTful web APIs so that independently developed apps can read and write data securely using OAuth 2.0 authorization and scoped access. The goal is to enable an app ecosystem rather than build bespoke interfaces for each vendor. Which standard is designed for this API-based, resource-oriented exchange?

A) HL7 Version 2.x
B) HL7 FHIR (Fast Healthcare Interoperability Resources)
C) HL7 CDA (Clinical Document Architecture)
D) EDI X12

Answer: B — HL7 FHIR (Fast Healthcare Interoperability Resources) represents clinical and administrative information as modular, independently addressable "resources" (Patient, Observation, MedicationRequest, and many more) exposed over RESTful APIs, and the SMART on FHIR profile layers OAuth 2.0 authorization and scopes on top, which is exactly the third-party app integration model described. FHIR's resource granularity and web-standard transport are why it underpins modern app ecosystems, certified-API requirements, and USCDI-based standardized API access in current federal rules. HL7 V2.x is message-based and event-driven, CDA is document-based and persistent, and X12 is EDI for batch administrative transactions; none of them provides FHIR's RESTful, resource-oriented API with OAuth 2.0 authorization and scopes. Because the architect's goal is an app marketplace with secure per-app read/write rather than custom interfaces, FHIR is uniquely suited and the alternatives are the wrong tool for the job.

Q13. At an annual board retreat, a CIO presents a document that links the organization's strategic goals—such as reducing readmissions and improving patient access—to specific IT initiatives, sequenced and resourced over a three-year horizon, with explicit dependencies, funding assumptions, and decision gates at which the organization can reassess. The board values it because it shows how technology spending will advance the mission rather than simply listing projects. This artifact is best described as which of the following?

A) A strategic IT plan
B) An incident response plan
C) A disaster recovery runbook
D) A data dictionary

Answer: A — A strategic IT plan translates enterprise strategic objectives—such as reducing readmissions and improving patient access—into a sequenced, resourced, multi-year set of IT initiatives with explicit dependencies and decision gates, ensuring that technology investments demonstrably advance the organization's mission and can be governed against milestones. This alignment artifact is the bridge between the organizational strategy and the project portfolio, and it is what governance bodies use to fund and stage initiatives over time. An incident response plan and a disaster recovery runbook address operational continuity and recovery from disruptions, and a data dictionary documents data element definitions and metadata; each is a legitimate and necessary artifact but operates at the tactical or operational level. None of them performs the multi-year strategic-alignment roadmap function the CIO is presenting to the board, so they are plausible-sounding distractors that fail the strategic-scope test.

Q14. A project manager is overseeing testing for a new clinical documentation system before go-live. Early in the cycle, the QA team executes test cases that confirm individual functions in isolation—verifying, for example, that a single order signs correctly and that a discrete field validates as designed—before any modules are combined. Later, the team verifies that the order-entry, pharmacy, and billing modules exchange data and work together correctly end-to-end across their interfaces. The first activity is unit/functional testing; the second activity, which validates that the separately built modules interoperate, is which type of testing?

A) Integration testing
B) Regression testing
C) Penetration testing
D) Smoke testing

Answer: A — Integration testing verifies that independently developed modules or systems interact correctly when combined, validating the data flow and interfaces across components—exactly the end-to-end order-to-pharmacy-to-billing scenario described after the individual functions passed unit testing. It sits between unit testing and system or user-acceptance testing in the SDLC verification sequence, catching defects in the seams—data mapping, interface formats, and timing—that unit testing cannot surface because it examines components in isolation. Regression testing confirms that new changes did not break previously working functionality, penetration testing probes security weaknesses, and smoke testing is a shallow build-acceptance check run before deeper testing begins. None of these is defined by verifying that separately built modules interoperate correctly, which is the defining purpose of integration testing and the precise activity the order-to-pharmacy-to-billing scenario describes.

Q15. A health system experiences a ransomware incident that encrypts its primary EHR database and forces a failover to downtime procedures. As the recovery team activates the disaster recovery plan, it references two predefined targets that were established during business impact analysis: the maximum tolerable amount of data loss measured backward in time from the moment of the incident, and the maximum tolerable downtime before the system must be restored to service. These two targets are, respectively:

A) MTBF and MTTR
B) SLA and OLA
C) RPO (recovery point objective) and RTO (recovery time objective)
D) KPI and KRI

Answer: C — The recovery point objective (RPO) defines the maximum acceptable amount of data loss measured backward in time from the disruption, which in turn dictates how frequently backups or replication must occur; the recovery time objective (RTO) defines the maximum acceptable downtime before the system must be restored to service. Together they drive backup frequency, replication architecture, and continuity investment, and they are central to any EHR disaster-recovery plan and the business impact analysis that precedes it. A short RPO demands more frequent backups or continuous replication, while a short RTO demands hot standby capacity—so the two targets shape very different parts of the recovery design. MTBF and MTTR are reliability and repair metrics, SLA and OLA are agreement types between provider and customer or between internal teams, and KPI and KRI are performance and risk indicators; none of these pairs defines the data-loss and downtime tolerances the recovery team is referencing.

Q16. A project sponsor must defend a proposed $1.2M enterprise analytics investment to the finance committee, which insists that benefits realized in future years be weighed against the cost of capital rather than counted at face value. The sponsor asks the project manager to quantify whether the investment is financially worthwhile by discounting the projected future cash flows back to present value using the organization's required rate of return and subtracting the initial outlay, where a positive result indicates the project creates value. Which metric is the sponsor requesting?

A) Net present value (NPV)
B) Total cost of ownership (TCO)
C) Break-even unit volume
D) Gross margin

Answer: A — Net present value (NPV) discounts a project's expected future cash inflows and outflows back to present value using a required rate of return (the discount rate) and subtracts the initial outlay; a positive NPV indicates the project is expected to create value, which is precisely the calculation the sponsor describes for the $1.2M analytics investment. NPV is generally preferred over payback period for capital decisions because it accounts for the time value of money across the entire benefit horizon rather than stopping at the recovery point, and it directly satisfies the finance committee's insistence on discounting. TCO enumerates lifecycle costs but says nothing about benefits, break-even unit volume is an operational throughput threshold, and gross margin is a profitability ratio. None of these performs the discounted-cash-flow valuation that NPV provides, so each is a distractor that measures a different financial dimension than the one the sponsor was asked to compute.

Q17. A privacy officer at a multi-facility health system is responding to an internal audit finding that several staff could view PHI well beyond what their duties required. She is implementing controls to ensure that each workforce member can access only the minimum protected health information necessary to perform their specific job functions, and she wants to pair an enforcement mechanism with the governing regulatory principle. Which combination of HIPAA-aligned access principles best operationalizes least-privilege access to PHI?

A) Shared generic accounts plus annual password rotation
B) Role-based access control plus the minimum necessary standard
C) Open access with retrospective audit only
D) Mandatory full-record access for all clinicians

Answer: B — Role-based access control (RBAC) assigns permissions according to defined job roles rather than to individuals ad hoc, and the HIPAA minimum necessary standard limits the use, disclosure, and request of PHI to what is reasonably needed for the task at hand; together they operationalize least-privilege access. Pairing RBAC with minimum necessary gives the privacy officer both an enforcement mechanism and the regulatory principle it serves, directly remediating the audit finding that staff could view PHI beyond their duties. Shared generic accounts defeat individual accountability and auditability, open access with retrospective audit detects but does not prevent inappropriate access, and mandatory full-record access for all clinicians directly violates minimum necessary by granting more than the role requires. Each alternative therefore weakens rather than enforces least privilege, which is why the RBAC-plus-minimum-necessary pairing is the only correct combination.

Q18. A program manager is evaluating two implementation strategies for a new EHR across a 12-hospital system with limited at-the-elbow support staff. Option 1 deploys to all twelve hospitals simultaneously on a single conversion date to minimize the period of running dual states. Option 2 deploys to one hospital first, stabilizes it and captures lessons learned, then proceeds hospital by hospital in successive waves. Option 1 is a "big bang" cutover. Option 2 is best described as which implementation strategy?

A) A parallel run
B) A pilot-only deployment
C) A phased (staggered/rolling) rollout
D) A canary release of code only

Answer: C — A phased (staggered or rolling) rollout deploys a system incrementally—here, one hospital at a time with a stabilization period between waves—which reduces the blast radius of any single failure and lets lessons learned in early waves improve configuration, training, and support for later ones. The trade-off versus a big-bang cutover is a longer overall timeline and a period during which the enterprise runs two states, but for a 12-hospital system with limited at-the-elbow support, that trade-off is usually worth the dramatic reduction in simultaneous risk. A parallel run operates the old and new systems concurrently to compare outputs, a pilot is a limited test that need not expand systemwide, and a canary release is a narrow software-deployment technique that exposes new code to a small slice of traffic. None of these matches the staggered, site-by-site go-live with stabilization between waves that Option 2 describes, so each is a distractor naming a different deployment concept.

Q19. A health system's IT leadership and its clinical business units have negotiated explicit performance commitments for the service desk—for example, "95% of priority-2 incidents resolved within 4 hours" and defined availability targets for core applications—along with the metrics, reporting cadence, and remedies that apply if targets are missed. The director needs to point to the single document that formally codifies these commitments between IT and the business units and serves as the basis for accountability. Which document is it?

A) A service-level agreement (SLA)
B) A business associate agreement (BAA)
C) A statement of work (SOW)
D) A request for proposal (RFP)

Answer: A — A service-level agreement (SLA) formally defines the agreed performance targets, metrics, responsibilities, reporting, and remedies between a service provider and its customer—precisely the "95% of priority-2 incidents resolved within 4 hours" commitment described—and provides the measurable basis for holding the service desk accountable. SLAs are commonly decomposed internally into operational-level agreements (OLAs) between supporting teams and supported by underpinning contracts with external suppliers, so that the customer-facing commitment is achievable end to end. A BAA governs PHI handling under HIPAA, an

SOW scopes deliverables, schedule, and acceptance criteria for a specific engagement, and an RFP solicits vendor proposals during procurement. None of these codifies the ongoing, measurable service performance targets that distinguish an SLA, which is why the SLA is the only correct fit for an enduring resolution-time commitment.

Q20. A health system's IT steering committee is frustrated that initiatives are approved one at a time by whichever executive sponsors them, leaving the organization overcommitted and out of alignment with strategy. Leadership wants to manage the full collection of active and proposed IT projects and programs as a coordinated whole—prioritizing, sequencing, and balancing them against resource capacity, risk, and strategic value rather than approving each request in isolation. This discipline is known as:

A) Incident management
B) Release management
C) Configuration management
D) Portfolio management

Answer: D — Portfolio management governs the organization's entire set of active and proposed programs and projects as a unified investment portfolio, prioritizing, sequencing, and balancing them against strategic objectives, resource capacity, and risk to maximize aggregate value rather than approving initiatives in isolation. It answers "are we doing the right projects?" at the enterprise level, complementing project management's "are we doing the projects right?" and directly addressing the steering committee's frustration with one-at-a-time, sponsor-driven approvals. Incident management restores service, release management deploys changes, and configuration management maintains accurate records of IT assets; all three are operational service-management disciplines focused on day-to-day delivery and stability rather than enterprise investment selection. None of them governs the coordinated, capacity-balanced, strategy-aligned prioritization of the full project set, which is the defining work of portfolio management.

Q21. A director is leading a major workflow change associated with rolling out computerized provider order entry (CPOE), a transition known historically to provoke significant clinician resistance. Rather than relying on the technology alone, she identifies key stakeholders and influencers, communicates a clear vision for why the change matters, secures visible executive sponsorship, designs role-based training, and builds in mechanisms to reinforce and sustain the new behaviors after go-live. This structured, people-centered approach is best categorized as:

A) Source code version control
B) Capacity planning
C) Data normalization
D) Organizational change management

Answer: D — Organizational change management is the structured discipline of preparing, supporting, and reinforcing people through a transition—stakeholder identification, vision communication, executive sponsorship, training, and reinforcement of new behaviors—to maximize adoption and minimize resistance, which is decisive for high-disruption initiatives like CPOE where clinician buy-in determines success. Models such as Prosci's ADKAR and Kotter's eight-step model formalize this work, and in health IT the human side of adoption is frequently the difference between a CPOE success and a costly failure or rollback. Source code version control tracks changes to software, capacity planning sizes infrastructure to demand, and data normalization organizes database structure to reduce redundancy; all three are technical activities that address software, infrastructure, and data design rather than people. None of them captures the stakeholder-, sponsorship-, training-, and reinforcement-focused approach the director is using, so each is a technical distractor offered against a behavioral-management answer.

Q22. A health system's compliance team is reviewing a complaint alleging that the organization unreasonably delayed sending a patient's records to a competing provider's app. The team must evaluate the conduct against the federal requirement that prohibits actors from engaging in practices likely to interfere with the access, exchange, or use of electronic health information, unless the practice satisfies one of the regulation's defined exceptions. Which regulatory provision are they addressing?

A) The HIPAA Privacy Rule's notice of privacy practices requirement
B) The Stark Law self-referral prohibition
C) The information-blocking rule under the 21st Century Cures Act
D) The Anti-Kickback Statute safe harbors

Answer: C — The 21st Century Cures Act's information-blocking provisions, implemented by ASTP/ONC, prohibit covered actors—health care providers, certified health IT developers, and health information networks/exchanges—from engaging in practices likely to interfere with the access, exchange, or use of electronic health information unless one of the defined exceptions (for example, preventing harm, privacy, security, or infeasibility) applies.

Compliance therefore turns on whether a given practice fits a defined exception, not on a blanket permission to withhold data, so the team must analyze the alleged delay against the specific exception criteria. The HIPAA notice-of-privacy-practices requirement governs how an entity informs patients about its data practices, while the Stark Law and Anti-Kickback Statute govern prohibited physician financial relationships and improper inducements respectively. None of those three addresses interference with the access, exchange, or use of electronic health information, so they are statutory distractors that, while real and important, do not apply to an information-blocking complaint.

Q23. A systems analyst is documenting the future-state requirements for a new revenue cycle system that must be delivered within a fixed budget and timeline. She produces a model showing the inputs, processes, outputs, and data stores, and—knowing not every requested feature can be funded in the first release—a separate prioritized list that classifies each requirement so stakeholders can negotiate scope. The classification sorts requirements into must-have, should-have, could-have, and won't-have-this-time categories. The prioritization technique she is applying is known as:

A) RACI assignment
B) MoSCoW prioritization
C) SWOT analysis
D) PERT estimation

Answer: B — MoSCoW prioritization classifies requirements into Must-have, Should-have, Could-have, and Won't-have-this-time categories, giving stakeholders a shared, explicit basis for scope decisions and trade-offs when time or budget is constrained—exactly the must-have-versus-nice-to-have distinction the analyst is drawing. It keeps negotiation focused on the few non-negotiable capabilities that must ship in the first release while parking lower-value items, which is essential when budget and timeline are fixed. RACI clarifies who is Responsible, Accountable, Consulted, and Informed for each task; SWOT assesses strengths, weaknesses, opportunities, and threats for strategic planning; and PERT estimates activity durations under uncertainty for scheduling. None of these classifies requirements by priority, so each is a distractor that names a real but unrelated technique—a roles tool, a strategy tool, and an estimation tool respectively—rather than the must/should/could/won't requirement-prioritization method the analyst applied.

Q24. A hospital must transmit a clinical summary to a referral partner at a transition of care. The summary must be a single, persistent, human-readable yet machine-parsable file—structured with a header that carries context (patient, author, encounter) and a body organized into coded sections such as problems, medications, and allergies—so the receiving clinician can both read it and have key data discretely imported. The interoperability lead needs to specify the HL7 standard purpose-built for this document-level exchange, the same one that underlies the Continuity of Care Document (CCD). Which HL7 standard is it?

A) HL7 Version 2.x ADT messaging
B) DICOM structured reporting
C) HL7 Clinical Document Architecture (CDA)
D) NCPDP Telecommunication standard

Answer: C — HL7 Clinical Document Architecture (CDA) defines the structure and semantics of a persistent clinical document—an XML file with a header for context and coded body sections for problems, medications, allergies, and the like—and it underpins the Continuity of Care Document (CCD) commonly exchanged at referral and transitions of care. CDA's combination of human readability and machine-parsable coding is exactly what the transition-of-care summary requires, letting the receiving clinician read the narrative while discretely importing structured problems and medications. HL7 V2.x carries discrete event messages rather than persistent documents, DICOM structured reporting conveys imaging findings, and the NCPDP Telecommunication standard serves real-time pharmacy claims adjudication. None of those three is a document-level clinical standard, so each is a distractor; CDA, as the basis of the CCD, is the purpose-built choice for the referral summary described.

Q25. A chief information security officer (CISO) is designing the security architecture for the EHR environment and presents the strategy to the risk committee. She explains that no single safeguard should be relied upon; instead, multiple independent, layered controls—network segmentation, encryption in transit and at rest, role-based access controls, and continuous monitoring—should protect information so that the failure or bypass of any one control still leaves the system protected by the others. This security design principle is called:

A) Single sign-on
B) Data minimization
C) Tokenization
D) Defense in depth

Answer: D — Defense in depth applies multiple independent, layered security controls—network segmentation, encryption, access controls, logging, and monitoring—so that if any single control fails, the remaining layers continue to protect the asset, reducing the chance that one point of failure leads to compromise. It is an architectural principle that directly addresses the CISO's stated goal of no single safeguard being decisive. Single sign-on is an authentication convenience that, if anything, concentrates rather than layers access; data minimization limits the data collected and retained; and tokenization substitutes sensitive values with non-sensitive surrogates. Each of these is a specific control or technique that might *participate* in a layered defense, but none of them is the overarching architectural principle of layering independent safeguards so that no single failure is decisive. Because the CISO is describing that very principle—multiple independent layers backstopping one another—defense in depth is the correct term and the others are component-level distractors.

Q26. A health system's CIO is evaluating a move of the enterprise data warehouse and downstream business-intelligence workloads from an aging on-premises appliance to a cloud platform-as-a-service (PaaS) analytics offering. During the security review, the CISO asks the team to document exactly which obligations the organization will continue to own after migration so they are not overlooked in budgeting and staffing. Under the cloud shared responsibility model for PaaS, which set of obligations remains the customer's responsibility rather than the cloud provider's?

A) Physical security of the data center, hypervisor patching, and underlying database engine patching
B) Data classification, identity and access management configuration, and securing the data the organization loads into the platform
C) Patching the managed runtime, maintaining the operating system, and replacing failed storage hardware
D) Networking fabric maintenance, load balancer firmware, and physical media destruction

Answer: B — In the PaaS model the provider manages the physical infrastructure, host operating system, virtualization layer, and the managed platform and runtime, while the customer always retains responsibility for its own data, data classification, and how identities and access are configured. The "customer responsibility" line shifts as you move from IaaS to PaaS to SaaS — under IaaS the customer still patches the guest OS and middleware, whereas under SaaS the provider manages nearly everything except data and access — but data governance and IAM configuration never transfer to the provider at any tier. For a senior IT leader, the practical takeaway is that adopting cloud does not outsource accountability for safeguarding PHI; the organization must still classify the data, configure least-privilege access, and enforce encryption and logging within the platform. Options A, C, and D list responsibilities the provider assumes under PaaS and would mislead leadership into under-resourcing the controls that remain the customer's duty. Management takeaway: write the responsibility matrix into the contract and the BAA, and staff the security team to own the customer-side controls before go-live.

Q27. A 600-bed academic medical center is preparing to deploy a machine-learning model that predicts sepsis risk from EHR data and pushes alerts to bedside nurses. The CMIO, wary of deploying a black box, wants an established governance framework that addresses AI trustworthiness throughout the model's lifecycle — establishing governance, mapping the context of use, measuring risk and performance, and managing the risk over time as the model and population evolve. Which framework is most directly designed for this purpose?

A) HITRUST CSF
B) NIST AI Risk Management Framework (AI RMF 1.0)
C) COBIT 2019
D) ISO 9001

Answer: B — The NIST AI Risk Management Framework (AI RMF 1.0, released January 2023) is purpose-built for managing risks of AI systems and is organized around four functions: Govern, Map, Measure, and Manage. Govern cuts across the other three to establish a culture of risk management; Map establishes context; Measure analyzes and tracks risk; and Manage prioritizes and acts on it. The framework directly addresses the trustworthiness characteristics of valid and reliable, safe, secure and resilient, accountable and transparent, explainable and interpretable, privacy-enhanced, and fair-with-harmful-bias-managed AI across the entire lifecycle. For a sepsis-prediction model this is exactly the right lens: it forces the organization to document intended use, monitor for performance degradation, and assign accountable owners. The AI RMF is voluntary and outcome-focused rather than prescriptive, which makes it adaptable to a clinical setting, and it is increasingly referenced alongside FDA expectations and the EU AI Act as the de facto starting point for healthcare AI governance. HITRUST CSF and COBIT 2019 address information security and enterprise IT governance broadly; ISO 9001 is a general quality-management standard — none is AI-lifecycle specific. Management takeaway: pair the AI RMF with a standing AI governance committee that signs off before any predictive model touches patient care.

Q28. A vendor's clinical decision-support software analyzes head CT imaging studies and autonomously flags suspected intracranial hemorrhage, moving those studies to the top of the radiologist's worklist and thereby driving a time-critical triage decision in which the clinician cannot independently re-derive the algorithm's basis in the moment. The organization's regulatory affairs lead is determining the correct U.S. oversight pathway before the tool goes live. Under FDA's framework, this product is most accurately characterized as:

A) A wellness device exempt from FDA oversight
B) Software as a Medical Device (SaMD) subject to FDA regulation
C) Certified Health IT regulated solely under ONC criteria
D) A laboratory-developed test regulated under CLIA

Answer: B — FDA, harmonizing with the International Medical Device Regulators Forum, defines Software as a Medical Device as software intended for one or more medical purposes that performs those purposes without being part of a hardware medical device. Autonomous detection of intracranial hemorrhage that drives a triage decision is a high-risk diagnostic and clinical-decision function meeting the device definition; it does not qualify for the non-device clinical-decision-support carve-out in the 21st Century Cures Act because the clinician cannot independently review the basis of the recommendation in the time-critical triage moment. Such products typically clear via the 510(k) or De Novo pathway, and FDA's evolving total-product-lifecycle and predetermined-change-control-plan approaches let manufacturers update the algorithm under an agreed protocol without a new submission for every change. ONC Health IT Certification governs EHR functionality and interoperability criteria, and CLIA governs the operation of clinical laboratories — neither is the primary regulatory pathway for this imaging-analysis algorithm, and option A wrongly assumes exemption. Management takeaway: confirm the FDA clearance status and intended-use statement of any diagnostic algorithm before clinical deployment, and track post-market performance as a condition of continued use.

Q29. A CFO and CIO are jointly deciding how to acquire a new enterprise scheduling platform, and the choice carries accounting consequences the board will scrutinize. One path is a perpetual software license installed on servers the organization buys and owns; the other is a multi-year cloud SaaS subscription billed monthly. Treating the acquisition as the SaaS subscription rather than the perpetual license with on-premises servers primarily shifts the spending from:

A) Operating expense (op-ex) to capital expense (cap-ex)
B) Capital expense (cap-ex) to operating expense (op-ex)
C) Direct cost to indirect cost with no cap-ex/op-ex effect
D) A sunk cost to an opportunity cost

Answer: B — Buying perpetual licenses and physical servers is a capital expenditure: a large up-front outlay capitalized on the balance sheet and depreciated over the asset's useful life. A SaaS subscription is consumed and expensed in the period incurred, making it operating expense with a smoother, predictable monthly run rate. This cap-ex-to-op-ex shift is one of the central financial trade-offs leaders weigh in cloud strategy because it affects cash flow timing, the balance sheet, depreciation schedules, and how the investment is approved and budgeted — op-ex often clears governance faster but accumulates indefinitely, while cap-ex requires capital-committee approval but ends once depreciated. Leaders also weigh that subscriptions transfer refresh and maintenance risk to the vendor but expose the organization to ongoing price increases and lock-in. A CIO must articulate this trade-off to the CFO rather than assume cloud is automatically cheaper. Management takeaway: model the multi-year cash-flow and balance-sheet impact, not just year-one cost, when choosing between perpetual licensing and subscription.

Q30. During systems-development-lifecycle planning for a new patient-portal release, the project manager must satisfy the governance board that the finished product actually meets the documented functional requirements and is fit for its intended use before it is promoted to production. The team prepares to execute a suite of test cases derived directly from those requirements to confirm the system does what it was specified to do. This phase is best described as:

A) Verification
B) Validation
C) Regression testing
D) Acceptance criteria definition

Answer: B — Validation answers "did we build the right system?" — confirming the finished product meets the user's actual requirements and intended use, typically through executing requirement-derived test cases and user-acceptance testing before production release. Verification ("did we build the system right?") is the complementary activity that checks conformance to specifications, design documents, and standards at each intermediate stage through reviews, inspections, and unit tests. Because the question specifies executing test cases derived directly from the functional requirements to confirm the system does what it was specified to do, validation is the precise term. Regression testing confirms that changes did not break previously working functionality, and acceptance-criteria definition is an upstream planning activity, not the execution phase described. Management takeaway: require traceability from each requirement to a validation test case so leadership can demonstrate coverage before sign-off.

Q31. A health system is adopting a zero-trust security architecture following a tabletop exercise that revealed an attacker could move laterally across the internal network once past the firewall. The CISO is briefing the executive team and must explain, in one sentence, what fundamentally changes under zero trust. Which statement best captures the core principle that distinguishes zero trust from a traditional perimeter-based model?

A) All traffic inside the corporate network is implicitly trusted once a user authenticates at the firewall
B) Trust is never implicit; every access request is continuously authenticated, authorized, and validated regardless of network location
C) A hardened network perimeter eliminates the need for internal segmentation and least-privilege controls
D) VPN connectivity alone is sufficient to grant trusted access to all internal resources

Answer: B — Zero trust, as articulated in NIST Special Publication 800-207, operates on "never trust, always verify": no user, device, or workload is granted implicit trust based on its network location, and every access request is continuously authenticated, authorized, and validated against identity, device posture, and contextual signals before access is granted, then re-evaluated throughout the session. This replaces the legacy "castle-and-moat" assumption that anything inside the corporate firewall is safe — an assumption that lets an attacker who breaches the perimeter move laterally at will, exactly the failure the tabletop exercise exposed. Zero trust instead relies on micro-segmentation, least-privilege access, continuous device-posture checks, and strong, often phishing-resistant authentication to shrink the blast radius of any single compromise. Options A, C, and D all restate the perimeter-trust assumptions that zero trust explicitly rejects, including the dangerous notion that a VPN alone confers trusted access. Management takeaway: treat zero trust as a multi-year architecture program anchored in identity and segmentation, not a single product purchase.

Q32. As part of business-continuity and disaster-recovery planning, an organization conducts a business-impact analysis with clinical leadership and sets formal recovery objectives for its EHR. Leadership determines that, after a major outage, the EHR must be restored to a working state within four hours, and that no more than fifteen minutes of transactional data may be lost. These two objectives will drive the failover design and the backup-and-replication frequency, respectively. The four-hour and fifteen-minute figures correspond, respectively, to:

A) RPO and RTO
B) RTO and RPO
C) MTD and MTTR
D) SLA and OLA

Answer: B — Recovery Time Objective (RTO) is the maximum acceptable duration to restore a system or service to operation after a disruption — here, four hours — and it drives investment in redundancy, failover, and recovery tooling. Recovery Point Objective (RPO) is the maximum acceptable amount of data loss measured in time — here, fifteen minutes — and it dictates how frequently backups or replication must run, since the organization can tolerate losing at most the last fifteen minutes of transactions. The figures in the stem therefore map to RTO then RPO. Maximum Tolerable Downtime (MTD), Mean Time To Repair (MTTR), Service Level Agreement (SLA), and Operating Level Agreement (OLA) are related continuity and service concepts but are not the two objectives matched to these specific values. Management takeaway: derive RTO and RPO from a business-impact analysis with clinical leadership, then fund replication and failover to meet them — never set them arbitrarily.

Q33. A health-IT department is performing a financial comparison of two competing infrastructure options for a new imaging archive. The first has a low purchase price but high annual support and energy costs; the second is more expensive up front but cheaper to run. Leadership insists the analysis include not just the purchase price but ongoing maintenance, staffing, power, training, downtime, and eventual decommissioning over the asset's life so the cheaper-to-buy option is not chosen by mistake. This comprehensive financial measure is known as:

A) Net present value (NPV)
B) Return on investment (ROI)

C) Total cost of ownership (TCO)
D) Internal rate of return (IRR)

Answer: C — Total cost of ownership captures all direct and indirect costs over the full lifecycle of an asset or solution — acquisition, implementation, integration, operation, staffing, power and facilities, training, downtime, maintenance, support, and eventual decommissioning — not just the initial sticker price. It is the discipline that prevents leaders from being seduced by a low purchase price that hides expensive ongoing costs, and it is essential when comparing on-premises versus cloud or one vendor versus another. In this scenario the lower-priced imaging archive may well lose to the costlier option once five years of support and energy are included. NPV and IRR are discounted-cash-flow valuation techniques that account for the time value of money, and ROI measures benefit relative to cost; TCO is specifically the comprehensive all-in lifecycle cost measure the question describes. Management takeaway: insist that vendor comparisons present TCO over the same multi-year horizon, since the lowest purchase price often carries the highest lifecycle cost.

Q34. A selection committee has already narrowed the field to three competing vendors for a new revenue-cycle platform after an earlier market-scan exercise. The requirements are now well understood, and the committee wants each vendor to submit a detailed, comparable response covering functional capabilities, pricing, implementation approach, support model, and client references so the responses can be scored side by side. To solicit these proposals, the committee should issue a:

A) Request for Information (RFI)
B) Request for Proposal (RFP)
C) Request for Quotation (RFQ)
D) Statement of Work (SOW)

Answer: B — A Request for Proposal solicits comprehensive, structured proposals from qualified vendors and is the appropriate instrument when the organization understands its requirements and wants comparable bids covering functional capabilities, implementation approach, pricing, support model, and references for a complex solution like a revenue-cycle platform. An RFI is an earlier, informational market-scan tool used to learn what solutions exist and shortlist vendors before requirements are fully defined; an RFQ is used to obtain price quotes on well-defined commodity items where price is the main variable; and a Statement of Work defines deliverables, milestones, and scope within an already-executed contract, not a competitive solicitation. The committee's need for detailed, comparable, multi-dimensional proposals points squarely to the RFP. Management takeaway: build the RFP scoring rubric and weights before proposals arrive to keep the evaluation objective and defensible.

Q35. A covered entity is finalizing a contract with a cloud vendor that will store and process protected health information on the covered entity's behalf, even though the vendor's staff will rarely if ever view the data directly. Procurement asks whether any specific agreement is legally required before the vendor may handle PHI. Under HIPAA, the parties must execute a:

A) Service-level agreement (SLA)
B) Business associate agreement (BAA)
C) Memorandum of understanding (MOU)
D) Data-use agreement (DUA) for limited data sets

Answer: B — A Business Associate Agreement is the HIPAA-required contract that obligates a business associate to safeguard PHI, restrict its use and disclosure to permitted purposes, implement appropriate administrative, physical, and technical safeguards, report security incidents and breaches, ensure subcontractors agree to the same terms, and comply with the applicable Privacy and Security Rule provisions. A cloud vendor that stores or processes PHI on behalf of the covered entity is a business associate even if it never views the data, so a signed BAA must be in place before any PHI is transmitted. An SLA defines performance and uptime metrics, an MOU is a typically non-binding statement of understanding, and a DUA governs limited data sets for research or public health — none of which substitutes for the BAA when a vendor handles identifiable PHI. Management takeaway: make an executed BAA a hard gate in procurement so no vendor can receive PHI before the agreement is signed.

Q36. A health system's EHR optimization project promised the board $4 million in annual savings and a measurable reduction in documentation time. Eighteen months after go-live, the board asks the CIO to demonstrate that those projected financial benefits and outcomes are actually being achieved and tracked rather than merely assumed. Which discipline most directly addresses measuring whether expected outcomes and value are realized over time?

A) Change-control management
B) Benefits realization management
C) Capacity planning

D) Configuration management

Answer: B — Benefits realization management is the structured practice of identifying, defining, planning, tracking, and measuring the expected benefits of an investment to ensure the projected value is actually delivered and sustained well after implementation. It closes the loop on the business case by defining baseline metrics, assigning benefit owners, and measuring outcomes over time — addressing the well-documented gap in which organizations approve projects on optimistic projections but never confirm whether the savings or quality gains materialized. Critically, benefits realization continues well past project closeout, since many EHR-optimization benefits accrue only after months of adoption and workflow stabilization. This is exactly what the board is asking the CIO to do. Change-control management governs how changes to systems are reviewed and approved, capacity planning ensures sufficient resources for demand, and configuration management tracks system component states — all operational disciplines that do not focus on tracking whether promised value was realized. Management takeaway: define baseline and target metrics and assign a benefit owner in the business case itself, then report realized benefits to the board on a fixed cadence.

Q37. Across a newly merged health system, two clinical applications each maintain their own patient demographic records, and a registration audit found thousands of duplicate and conflicting patient identities — some patients appear two or three times with slightly different spellings and birth dates, creating safety and billing risk. The CIO wants a single authoritative, governed source for patient identity data that is shared and reconciled across all systems. The most appropriate solution is:

A) An extract-transform-load (ETL) batch job run nightly
B) A master data management (MDM) program with an enterprise master patient index
C) A data lake storing all raw source records
D) A reporting data mart for the registration department

Answer: B — Master data management establishes governed, authoritative "golden records" for the critical shared entities an enterprise depends on — patients, providers, locations, payers — and in healthcare it is typically realized through an enterprise master patient index that matches, links, and de-duplicates patient identities across source systems using deterministic and probabilistic matching. This directly solves the duplicate-and-conflicting-identity problem described and provides a single authoritative source other systems can reference. ETL moves and transforms data but does not by itself create or steward an authoritative identity; a data lake stores raw source records without resolving conflicts or enforcing governance; and a reporting data mart serves analytics for a single department rather than enterprise identity stewardship. In a post-merger context the EMPI is especially valuable because it reconciles the legacy identity domains of both organizations into one trusted index. Only MDM with an EMPI delivers the governed single source of truth the CIO requires. Management takeaway: pair the EMPI with data-stewardship roles and a duplicate-resolution workflow, since matching technology without governance still drifts back into duplicates.

Q38. A CISO has been asked by the board to benchmark the organization's cybersecurity maturity using a widely adopted, sector-neutral, outcome-based framework that lets leadership compare a current profile against a target profile in plain business language. The framework is organized around six core functions: Govern, Identify, Protect, Detect, Respond, and Recover. This describes:

A) NIST Cybersecurity Framework (CSF) 2.0
B) PCI DSS
C) HIPAA Security Rule administrative safeguards
D) ISO/IEC 20000

Answer: A — The NIST Cybersecurity Framework 2.0, released in 2024, organizes cybersecurity outcomes into six core functions: Govern, Identify, Protect, Detect, Respond, and Recover. The newly added Govern function — which establishes and monitors the organization's cybersecurity risk-management strategy, expectations, and policy — is what distinguishes CSF 2.0 from version 1.1, which had only the original five functions. The framework is outcome-based and voluntary, allowing organizations to map their current and target profiles regardless of sector. PCI DSS targets payment-card data security, the HIPAA Security Rule prescribes specific required and addressable safeguards for ePHI, and ISO/IEC 20000 is an IT service-management standard — none of these is organized around the six CSF functions named in the stem. Management takeaway: use CSF profiles to communicate current-versus-target maturity to the board in plain language and to prioritize the security roadmap.

Q39. Persistent physician complaints about EHR usability and a stalled CPOE adoption effort have convinced senior leadership that the IT organization lacks credible clinical leadership. They decide to create a single accountable executive role to define the clinical informatics strategy, champion physician adoption of the EHR, and serve as the primary bridge between the medical staff and the IT organization. Which role most appropriately fills this responsibility?

A) Chief Information Security Officer (CISO)
B) Chief Medical Informatics Officer (CMIO)
C) Chief Financial Officer (CFO)
D) Chief Nursing Officer (CNO)

Answer: B — The Chief Medical Informatics Officer (sometimes titled Chief Medical Information Officer) is the physician executive who leads clinical informatics strategy, drives physician engagement with and adoption of clinical systems such as the EHR and CPOE, and serves as the essential translator between the medical staff and the IT organization. Because the CMIO is a practicing or formerly practicing physician, this role carries the clinical credibility needed to champion workflow change and reduce physician burnout from poorly designed systems. The CISO owns information security, the CFO owns finance, and the Chief Nursing Officer leads nursing practice broadly; the analogous nursing-informatics bridge role would be the CNIO. The specific responsibility of bridging the medical staff and IT belongs to the CMIO. Management takeaway: give the CMIO real authority over clinical-system design decisions, not just an advisory title, to make physician adoption stick.

Q40. A data-science team has moved beyond pilots and is now operationalizing several predictive models in production across the enterprise. After one model's accuracy quietly degraded when the patient mix shifted, leadership mandates disciplined processes for versioning models and their training data, automated retraining pipelines, continuous monitoring for performance and data drift, and controlled, reversible deployment. The set of practices that addresses these needs is collectively called:

A) DevSecOps
B) MLOps
C) ITIL incident management
D) Agile sprint planning

Answer: B — MLOps (machine-learning operations) extends DevOps principles to the machine-learning lifecycle, covering model and data versioning, reproducible and automated training pipelines, controlled deployment with rollback, and — critically for clinical models — ongoing monitoring for model performance degradation and data or concept drift that can silently erode accuracy as patient populations and practice patterns change. The needs listed in the stem map directly onto MLOps capabilities. DevSecOps integrates security earlier into the software-delivery pipeline but is not specific to the model lifecycle; ITIL incident management governs the handling of service disruptions; and Agile sprint planning organizes iterative software delivery — none addresses the versioning, retraining, drift-monitoring, and model-deployment concerns the team is operationalizing. Management takeaway: budget for MLOps tooling and ongoing monitoring at deployment time, because an unmonitored clinical model is a latent patient-safety risk.

Q41. A capital committee is comparing two IT investments, each with benefits and costs spread unevenly across five years, and must choose using a method that accounts for the time value of money rather than simple totals. To decide which project creates more value in today's dollars, leadership discounts each project's future cash flows to the present using the organization's cost of capital and subtracts the initial outlay. Under this approach, a project should generally be considered financially acceptable when its:

A) Payback period exceeds the asset's useful life
B) Net present value (NPV) is greater than zero
C) Total cost of ownership equals its purchase price
D) ROI is negative but the IRR is high

Answer: B — Net present value discounts all projected future cash inflows and outflows to present value using a required rate of return (the discount rate) and subtracts the initial investment; a positive NPV means the project is expected to generate returns exceeding the organization's cost of capital and therefore creates value, making it financially acceptable. When comparing two projects, the one with the higher positive NPV generally creates more value in today's dollars, and unlike simple payback NPV properly credits benefits that arrive in later years while discounting them for risk and the time value of money. A payback period longer than the asset's useful life is unfavorable, total cost of ownership measures lifecycle cost rather than value creation, and a negative ROI signals the project does not even return its cost — so option B is the correct acceptance test. Management takeaway: pair NPV with sensitivity analysis on the discount rate and benefit assumptions so the capital committee understands the range of outcomes, not a single point estimate.

Q42. Eighteen months into a multi-cloud strategy, an organization finds its monthly cloud spend rising unpredictably as engineering teams provision resources independently with little visibility into who is spending what. Finance and IT are pointing fingers, and the original business case is eroding. Leadership wants a cross-functional discipline that brings shared financial accountability to cloud consumption — combining real-time cost visibility, allocation and showback, rightsizing, and continuous optimization. This practice is known as:

A) FinOps
B) GreenOps
C) Capital budgeting
D) Activity-based costing

Answer: A — FinOps (cloud financial operations) is the cultural and operational discipline that brings financial accountability to the variable-spend model of cloud, uniting finance, engineering, and business teams so they can gain near-real-time cost visibility, allocate and show back or charge back spend to the consuming teams, rightsize and schedule resources, leverage commitment-based discounts, and continuously optimize. It is purpose-built for the unpredictable, consumption-based nature of cloud billing in which decentralized teams provision resources on demand. Capital budgeting and activity-based costing are general financial methods that predate cloud and do not provide the continuous, cross-functional cloud-cost governance described, and GreenOps focuses on environmental sustainability rather than financial accountability. Management takeaway: stand up a cross-functional FinOps practice with showback dashboards early in a cloud journey, before unmanaged consumption erodes the business case.

Q43. During vendor risk management for a new SaaS analytics platform that will hold de-identified and limited patient data, the security team must satisfy internal audit that the vendor's controls are not just well designed on paper but actually operating effectively over time. The team wants independent third-party assurance covering security, availability, and confidentiality across a defined audit period. The most relevant artifact to request is:

A) A SOC 2 Type II report
B) A SOC 1 Type I report
C) The vendor's marketing white paper
D) A signed nondisclosure agreement

Answer: A — A SOC 2 Type II report provides an independent CPA firm's opinion on both the design and the operating effectiveness of a service organization's controls assessed over a period of time (typically six to twelve months), evaluated against the AICPA Trust Services Criteria of security, availability, processing integrity, confidentiality, and privacy. This is exactly the period-of-time, design-and-operating-effectiveness assurance the security team wants for vendor risk management. A SOC 1 report addresses internal controls over financial reporting and is irrelevant to security assurance, while a Type I report covers only the design of controls at a single point in time and says nothing about whether they operated effectively across the audit period — which is precisely what internal audit demanded here. Marketing white papers and a signed NDA provide no independent control assurance whatsoever. Management takeaway: require a current SOC 2 Type II as a standing condition of vendor onboarding and renewal, and review the exceptions noted in the report rather than just confirming one exists.

Q44. A CIO is building the enterprise analytics roadmap and wants to distinguish the levels of analytic maturity so the organization invests in the right capabilities in the right order. Consider a dashboard that lets analysts explain *why* readmissions rose last quarter by drilling from the headline rate into contributing factors such as payer mix, discharge timing, and follow-up gaps to surface root causes. This capability represents which type of analytics?

A) Descriptive analytics
B) Diagnostic analytics
C) Predictive analytics
D) Prescriptive analytics

Answer: B — Diagnostic analytics answers "why did it happen?" by drilling into data to identify the contributing factors, correlations, and root causes behind an observed outcome — exactly the activity of explaining why readmissions rose by examining the drivers. The four-stage analytic maturity model proceeds from descriptive analytics ("what happened," e.g., the readmission rate itself), to diagnostic ("why did it happen"), to predictive ("what is likely to happen," e.g., which patients are at risk), to prescriptive ("what should we do," e.g., recommended interventions). Each stage adds value and complexity. Because the dashboard explains causation rather than merely reporting the number or forecasting future cases, it represents the diagnostic level. Management takeaway: sequence analytics investments up the maturity curve, since prescriptive value depends on first having trustworthy descriptive and diagnostic foundations.

Q45. After analysts repeatedly produced conflicting numbers for the same metric in board reports because no one agreed on definitions or ownership, a health system charters a data-governance council to establish enterprise policies for data quality, stewardship, common definitions, and accountability across all clinical and financial data domains. A skeptical executive asks the CIO to explain, in one sentence, what data governance actually is. Which statement best describes the primary purpose of data governance?

A) To purchase and maintain the physical storage hardware for the data warehouse
B) To establish the people, policies, processes, and standards that ensure data is accurate, consistent, secure, and used appropriately as an enterprise asset
C) To write the SQL queries that populate operational dashboards
D) To negotiate the licensing terms with the BI software vendor

Answer: B — Data governance is the exercise of authority, control, and shared decision-making over the management of data assets. It establishes the people (such as a governance council, data owners, and data stewards), policies, processes, standards, and definitions that ensure data is accurate, consistent, secure, well-defined, and used appropriately and ethically as a strategic enterprise asset. The chartered council's purpose to set enterprise policies for data quality, stewardship, definitions, and accountability is the essence of governance. It is fundamentally an organizational and policy discipline — not the procurement of storage hardware (A), the writing of dashboard queries (C), or the negotiation of software licensing (D), all of which are downstream technical or commercial tasks that governance may inform but does not consist of. Management takeaway: secure executive sponsorship and clear decision rights for the governance council up front, or its policies will be ignored by the operational teams.

Q46. A negotiated SLA for a hosted clinical application guarantees 99.9% monthly availability with financial credits payable to the health system for breaches. The operations director is uneasy because clinicians depend on the application around the clock and wants to translate the marketing figure into a concrete downtime budget before signing. A 99.9% monthly uptime SLA permits approximately how much unplanned downtime per month?

A) About 4 hours
B) About 43 minutes
C) About 8 hours
D) About 5 minutes

Answer: B — For a roughly 30-day month of about 43,200 minutes, 0.1 percent of allowable downtime (the complement of 99.9 percent) equals approximately 43 minutes. "Three nines" therefore tolerates only about 43 minutes of unplanned outage per month, which is why the next tier up, 99.99 percent or "four nines," permits only about 4 minutes per month and costs substantially more to engineer and operate. By contrast, 99 percent ("two nines") would allow more than seven hours of monthly downtime — unacceptable for a clinical system clinicians use around the clock. A senior leader must translate marketing "nines" into a concrete downtime budget to judge whether the guarantee matches the clinical criticality of the application and to size the financial credits appropriately. Option A (4 hours) corresponds to roughly 99.4 percent, option C (8 hours) to about 98.9 percent, and option D (5 minutes) to nearly four nines — none matches 99.9 percent. Management takeaway: negotiate SLA tiers to the clinical criticality of each application, and ensure the financial credits are large enough to matter rather than token amounts that the vendor treats as a cost of doing business.

Q47. A health system suffered a ransomware incident in which the attacker encrypted not only production systems but also the backup servers, because those backups were kept online and network-reachable from the same domain. Recovery took weeks and nearly forced a ransom payment. As part of the post-incident review, the CISO must recommend a backup-architecture change that prevents a future attacker from destroying the recovery copies. The most effective improvement is to:

A) Increase the RPO so fewer backups are required
B) Maintain immutable and/or air-gapped (offline) backup copies isolated from the production network
C) Store all backups on the same SAN as production for faster restores
D) Reduce backup frequency to limit attack surface

Answer: B — Ransomware increasingly targets connected, network-reachable backups precisely so victims cannot recover without paying, so resilient designs keep at least one copy immutable (write-once, retention-locked, tamper-resistant) and/or air-gapped and offline so it cannot be reached, encrypted, or deleted by an attacker who has compromised the production environment. This reflects the modern 3-2-1-1-0 backup strategy: three copies, on two media types, one off-site, one offline or immutable, with zero recovery errors verified by regular restore testing. The isolated copy is the organization's last line of defense against being forced to pay a ransom. Increasing the RPO (A) and reducing backup frequency (D) simply allow more data loss and do nothing to protect the backups themselves, and co-locating backups on the same production SAN (C) leaves them fully exposed to the very attack that took down production. Only immutable or air-gapped isolation addresses the failure mode described. Management takeaway: test restores from the isolated copy on a regular schedule, because an untested backup is only a hope, not a recovery capability.

Q48. A program manager is preparing the go/no-go evaluation for a new AI-enabled clinical documentation tool ahead of broad rollout across the medical group. The vendor has supplied impressive accuracy figures from its own validation, and standard functional and integration testing has passed. Beyond that conventional testing, which evaluation activity is most critical and distinctive for an AI/ML clinical tool before approving deployment?

A) Confirming the user-interface color palette meets brand guidelines
B) Validating model performance against representative clinical data, assessing bias/fairness across patient subgroups, and monitoring for drift after deployment
C) Verifying that the vendor's invoice matches the purchase order
D) Ensuring the login screen loads in under two seconds

Answer: B — AI and machine-learning clinical tools require evaluation specific to their probabilistic, data-driven nature: validating performance metrics such as sensitivity, specificity, positive predictive value, and calibration against representative local clinical data; assessing for algorithmic bias and inequitable performance across patient subgroups defined by race, sex, age, or payer; and establishing post-deployment monitoring for data drift and concept drift that can silently degrade accuracy once the model meets a population different from its training set. These are distinctive safety and equity risks not surfaced by conventional functional, integration, or performance testing, and impressive vendor-reported numbers from a different population are not a substitute for local validation. Verifying the UI color palette (A), matching the invoice to the purchase order (C), and confirming login speed (D) are ordinary procurement or usability checks unrelated to the model's clinical validity, fairness, and ongoing safety. Management takeaway: validate AI tools on the organization's own patient population before rollout, since vendor-reported metrics from a different population may not generalize.

Q49. A CIO is restructuring IT leadership after an audit criticized the prior arrangement, in which the same executive was responsible for both keeping systems running and securing them — a conflict that suppressed bad security news. The CIO wants responsibility for protecting the confidentiality, integrity, and availability of information assets — including security policy, enterprise risk management, and incident response — to rest with a single accountable executive who reports independently of the team running day-to-day operations. This role is the:

A) Chief Nursing Informatics Officer (CNIO)
B) Chief Information Security Officer (CISO)
C) Chief Technology Officer (CTO)
D) Chief Data Officer (CDO)

Answer: B — The Chief Information Security Officer is the senior executive singularly accountable for the organization's information-security program — setting security strategy and policy, leading enterprise risk management, overseeing the security operations center and incident response, and protecting the confidentiality, integrity, and availability (the classic CIA triad) of information assets. Positioning the CISO with reporting independence from the day-to-day IT operations team preserves objectivity and avoids the conflict of interest that arises when the same leader is judged on both uptime and security. The Chief Nursing Informatics Officer leads nursing informatics, the Chief Technology Officer leads technology architecture and infrastructure operations, and the Chief Data Officer leads data strategy and governance — none of which is the accountable owner of the information-security program described. Management takeaway: give the CISO a direct line to the board or audit committee so security risk is reported without being filtered through the operations leaders being assessed.

Q50. A health-IT steering committee faces twenty-two competing project requests for the coming fiscal year but a fixed annual capital budget that can fund perhaps eight of them. Department heads are lobbying hard, and the committee wants a defensible, repeatable way to decide that aligns selection with organizational strategy and ensures scarce funds go to the highest-value initiatives rather than the loudest sponsors. The most appropriate governance practice is to:

A) Fund projects strictly in the order the requests were submitted
B) Apply a structured portfolio-management process that scores and ranks projects against strategic alignment, expected value/ROI, risk, and resource capacity
C) Let each department fund whatever it wants from its own discretionary budget
D) Approve every project that has executive sponsorship regardless of cost

Answer: B — IT portfolio management applies a structured, repeatable, and transparent process to evaluate, score, and prioritize competing investments against explicit criteria such as strategic alignment, expected value or ROI, risk, regulatory necessity, and resource and capacity constraints — ensuring that a fixed pool of capital is directed to the highest-value initiatives and that the overall mix balances run, grow, and transform investments. This governance discipline gives the steering committee a defensible, repeatable basis for its decisions. Funding strictly by submission order (A), allowing uncoordinated departmental spending (C), and approving anything with an executive sponsor regardless of cost (D) all bypass strategic prioritization, reward politics over value, and lead to misallocated capital, redundant systems, and a fragmented portfolio over time. Management takeaway: publish the prioritization criteria and the resulting ranked list so declined requests are understood as a portfolio trade-off rather than a personal rejection.

.44 Glossary of Key Terms

Agile. An iterative software development and project management approach that delivers work in short increments (sprints), emphasizing adaptive planning, continuous stakeholder feedback, and frequent releases. CPHIMS candidates must contrast Agile with waterfall and recognize that hybrid models are common in regulated healthcare IT environments where validation and documentation requirements persist.

AI Governance. The organizational structures, policies, and oversight mechanisms that ensure artificial intelligence and machine learning systems are deployed safely, ethically, and in compliance with regulation. In healthcare, AI governance addresses model validation, bias monitoring, transparency, clinical oversight, and lifecycle management; senior IT leaders are expected to establish committees and accountability frameworks rather than treat AI as an ungoverned procurement.

API-First. A design philosophy in which application programming interfaces are treated as primary, contractually defined products built before or alongside the user interface, enabling modular integration and reuse. In health IT, an API-first strategy underpins modern interoperability, supporting FHIR-based exchange and reducing dependence on brittle point-to-point interfaces.

Application Portfolio. The complete inventory of software applications an organization owns or licenses, assessed for business value, technical health, cost, and redundancy. Portfolio rationalization—retiring, consolidating, or modernizing applications—is a core senior responsibility for controlling total cost and reducing technical debt.

Architecture Review Board (ARB). A governance body that evaluates proposed solutions, integrations, and technology selections against enterprise architecture standards and principles. The ARB enforces consistency, manages exceptions, and prevents the proliferation of incompatible or redundant systems across the enterprise.

Benefits Realization. The discipline of defining, measuring, and confirming the tangible and intangible value an IT investment was expected to deliver, tracked through and beyond go-live. Healthcare benefits realization links system adoption to outcomes such as reduced length of stay, improved quality scores, or labor savings, and is central to justifying continued investment.

Business Associate Agreement (BAA). A HIPAA-mandated contract between a covered entity and a vendor (business associate) that handles protected health information on its behalf, specifying permitted uses, safeguards, and breach-notification obligations. Senior IT leaders must ensure a BAA is executed before any third party touches PHI, including cloud and AI vendors.

Business Case. A structured justification for an investment that articulates the problem, options analyzed, costs, benefits, risks, and recommended course of action. Exam-relevant business cases integrate financial metrics (ROI, NPV, TCO) with strategic alignment and are the gating artifact before project funding.

Business Continuity / Disaster Recovery (BC/DR). A combined planning discipline ensuring critical business functions continue (BC) and IT systems are restored (DR) during and after a disruption. Healthcare BC/DR must address downtime procedures for clinical systems, with plans tested regularly and aligned to defined recovery objectives.

Build vs. Buy. The strategic decision between developing a custom solution internally and acquiring a commercial or cloud-based product. The analysis weighs cost, time-to-value, maintenance burden, differentiation, and risk; in healthcare the strong default is "buy/configure" given regulatory, support, and interoperability demands.

Capability Roadmap. A time-phased plan that maps how an organization's business and technical capabilities will evolve, sequencing initiatives to deliver strategic outcomes. It translates the IT strategic plan into a prioritized, dependency-aware schedule that communicates direction to stakeholders.

Change Management. The structured approach to preparing, equipping, and supporting people through organizational and technology transitions to achieve adoption and minimize disruption. Distinct from technical change control, this people-side discipline (often using models such as ADKAR or Kotter) is a frequent cause of healthcare IT project failure when neglected.

Chief Information Officer (CIO). The senior executive accountable for an organization's information technology strategy, operations, governance, and value delivery. The healthcare CIO aligns IT investments with clinical and business strategy and increasingly partners with clinical informatics and security leadership.

Chief Information Security Officer (CISO). The executive responsible for the enterprise information security and cybersecurity program, including risk management, policy, incident response, and compliance. In healthcare the CISO leads HIPAA Security Rule compliance, manages threats such as ransomware, and reports risk posture to executive leadership and the board.

Chief Medical Information Officer (CMIO). A physician leader who bridges clinical practice and information technology, guiding electronic health record optimization, clinical decision support, and physician adoption. The CMIO ensures technology decisions reflect clinical workflow and patient-safety priorities.

Chief Nursing Information Officer (CNIO). A nurse executive who represents nursing workflow, documentation, and adoption needs in health IT strategy and system design. The CNIO partners with the CMIO and CIO to ensure systems support frontline nursing practice and quality outcomes.

COBIT. A governance and management framework (Control Objectives for Information and Related Technologies, from ISACA) that aligns IT with enterprise goals through defined objectives, processes, and performance metrics. COBIT 2019 emphasizes governance versus management separation and is referenced for IT control, audit, and value delivery.

Critical Path. The longest sequence of dependent activities in a project schedule that determines the minimum project duration; any delay on this path delays the entire project. Senior project oversight focuses resources and risk attention on critical-path tasks to protect the timeline.

Data Governance. The framework of policies, roles, standards, and processes that ensure data is accurate, secure, available, and used appropriately across the enterprise. In healthcare it covers data quality, stewardship, master data, privacy, and regulatory reporting, and is foundational to analytics and AI initiatives.

Data Lakehouse. A modern data architecture that combines the low-cost, flexible storage of a data lake with the structured query, governance, and transactional reliability of a data warehouse. It enables organizations to support both analytics and machine learning on diverse healthcare data without maintaining fully separate platforms.

Data Warehouse. A centralized repository optimized for reporting and analysis, integrating data from multiple source systems into a consistent, historical, query-friendly structure. Enterprise data warehouses underpin clinical, operational, and financial analytics and quality reporting in healthcare organizations.

Demand Management. The process of capturing, evaluating, and prioritizing incoming requests for IT projects and services against available capacity and strategic priorities. Effective demand management prevents resource overload, surfaces redundant requests, and ensures the portfolio reflects organizational priorities.

Electronic Clinical Quality Measure (eCQM). A standardized quality measure that uses structured EHR data to assess care processes and outcomes for regulatory and value-based reporting programs. CPHIMS candidates must understand how eCQMs are specified, captured, and submitted, and how data-capture gaps affect reported performance.

Enterprise Architecture (EA). The holistic discipline of analyzing, designing, and governing an organization's business processes, information, applications, and technology infrastructure as an integrated whole. EA aligns IT capabilities with strategy, reduces complexity and redundancy, and provides the blueprint for transformation.

ETL. Extract, Transform, Load—the process of pulling data from source systems, converting it to a target format and structure, and loading it into a destination such as a data warehouse. Variants such as ELT (load before transform) are common in cloud and lakehouse architectures; senior leaders evaluate data-pipeline reliability and latency.

FHIR Bulk Data. A specification (the "Flat FHIR" or Bulk Data Access standard) that enables efficient export of large volumes of FHIR resources for populations of patients, supporting analytics, research, and quality reporting. It complements transactional FHIR APIs by serving population-scale rather than single-patient use cases.

FinOps. A cultural and operational practice for managing and optimizing cloud spending through cross-functional collaboration among finance, engineering, and business teams. As healthcare migrates workloads to the cloud, FinOps disciplines (visibility, allocation, optimization) help senior leaders control variable, consumption-based costs.

Go-Live. The milestone at which a new or upgraded system transitions into production use by end users, often supported by command centers, at-the-elbow support, and contingency plans. Healthcare go-lives are high-risk events requiring cutover planning, downtime procedures, and intensive change management.

Health Information Exchange (HIE). Both the act of electronically sharing health information across organizations and the entities or networks that facilitate that exchange. HIEs improve care coordination and population health; they are increasingly governed by national frameworks such as TEFCA.

HIPAA Security Rule. The federal regulation establishing required administrative, physical, and technical safeguards to protect the confidentiality, integrity, and availability of electronic protected health information. It mandates a risk-analysis–based, scalable approach to safeguards, with senior leaders accountable for compliance and documentation.

HL7 FHIR. Fast Healthcare Interoperability Resources, a modern interoperability standard from HL7 that represents clinical and administrative data as modular, web-friendly resources exchanged via RESTful APIs. FHIR (Release 4 and the R5 line, with US Core profiles) is the foundation of current U.S. interoperability policy and app ecosystems.

IT Steering Committee. A cross-functional executive body that prioritizes IT investments, approves major projects, and aligns the IT portfolio with organizational strategy. It provides the governance forum where competing demands are reconciled against budget and strategic objectives.

IT Strategic Plan. A multi-year roadmap that aligns information technology direction, investments, and capabilities with the organization's mission and business strategy. It establishes priorities, guiding principles, and measurable objectives, and serves as the anchor for portfolio and budget decisions.

ITIL. A widely adopted framework for IT service management that defines best practices for delivering and supporting IT services across their lifecycle. ITIL 4 emphasizes value streams, the service value system, and practices such as incident, problem, and change management relevant to healthcare IT operations.

Master Data Management (MDM). The discipline and technology for creating and maintaining a single, authoritative source of truth for key data entities such as patients, providers, and locations. In healthcare, enterprise master patient index and provider data management reduce duplicates and improve data integrity across systems.

MLOps. The set of practices that operationalize machine learning models—covering development, deployment, monitoring, retraining, and governance—analogous to DevOps for software. Healthcare MLOps must address model drift, validation, and regulatory expectations so that deployed AI remains safe and effective over time.

NIST AI Risk Management Framework (AI RMF). A voluntary framework from the National Institute of Standards and Technology that guides organizations in identifying, measuring, and managing risks of AI systems through four functions: Govern, Map, Measure, and Manage. It provides senior leaders a structured approach to trustworthy and responsible AI adoption.

NIST Cybersecurity Framework (CSF). A risk-based framework organizing cybersecurity activities into core functions—Govern, Identify, Protect, Detect, Respond, and Recover (Govern added in CSF 2.0). It offers a common language for assessing and improving security posture and is widely mapped to HIPAA requirements in healthcare.

Net Present Value (NPV). A financial metric that discounts a project's projected future cash flows to present-day value and subtracts the initial investment; a positive NPV indicates value creation. NPV accounts for the time value of money and is preferred over simple payback for comparing long-horizon IT investments.

Project Charter. A formal document that authorizes a project, defines its objectives, scope, key stakeholders, high-level budget, and the authority of the project manager. The charter is the foundational governance artifact that initiates a project and aligns sponsor expectations.

Project Portfolio Management (PPM). The centralized coordination and prioritization of projects and programs as a portfolio to optimize value, balance risk, and align with strategy under resource constraints. PPM gives senior leaders visibility to select, sequence, and govern initiatives rather than manage projects in isolation.

Qualified Health Information Network (QHIN). An entity designated under TEFCA that connects to other QHINs to enable nationwide health information exchange under a common agreement and technical framework. QHINs form the backbone of the TEFCA "network of networks," and leaders evaluate participation as part of interoperability strategy.

RACI. A responsibility-assignment matrix that clarifies who is Responsible, Accountable, Consulted, and Informed for each task or decision in a project or process. RACI prevents role ambiguity and is a standard governance tool for complex, cross-functional healthcare IT initiatives.

Recovery Point Objective (RPO). The maximum acceptable amount of data loss measured in time, defining how far back in time recovery must reach after a disruption. RPO drives backup frequency and replication design; clinical systems typically demand a low RPO to avoid losing patient data.

Recovery Time Objective (RTO). The maximum acceptable duration to restore a system or process after an outage before unacceptable consequences occur. RTO informs DR architecture and investment; critical clinical applications require short RTOs supported by redundancy and tested recovery procedures.

Regression Testing. The practice of re-running tests after changes, upgrades, or fixes to confirm that existing functionality still works as intended. In healthcare IT, regression testing is essential after EHR updates and interface changes to protect patient safety and avoid introducing defects.

Request for Proposal (RFP). A formal procurement document soliciting detailed vendor proposals against defined functional, technical, security, and contractual requirements. A well-structured RFP enables objective, weighted evaluation and supports defensible, governance-aligned vendor selection.

Return on Investment (ROI). A financial metric expressing the net benefit of an investment as a percentage of its cost, used to compare and justify initiatives. Healthcare ROI analyses should incorporate both hard savings and quantifiable quality or risk-reduction benefits while acknowledging non-financial value.

Risk Analysis. The systematic process of identifying, assessing, and prioritizing threats and vulnerabilities to information assets, including the likelihood and impact of potential security incidents. A documented, ongoing risk analysis is explicitly required by the HIPAA Security Rule and is the foundation for safeguard decisions.

Service Level Agreement (SLA). A contractual commitment defining the level of service a provider will deliver, including measurable targets for availability, performance, and support response, plus remedies for non-compliance. SLAs are central to vendor and cloud management and must reflect the criticality of healthcare systems.

Software as a Medical Device (SaMD). Software intended for one or more medical purposes that performs those purposes without being part of a hardware medical device, and is therefore subject to regulatory oversight (e.g., FDA). Senior leaders must recognize when clinical decision-support or AI software meets the SaMD definition, triggering regulatory and validation obligations.

Software Development Life Cycle (SDLC). The structured set of phases—such as planning, analysis, design, build, test, deploy, and maintain—through which software systems are developed and managed. Understanding SDLC models (waterfall, iterative, Agile) and their governance and validation implications is essential for managing healthcare system delivery.

Total Cost of Ownership (TCO). The comprehensive estimate of all direct and indirect costs of acquiring, operating, maintaining, and eventually retiring a system over its full lifecycle. TCO analysis prevents underestimating ongoing costs—licensing, infrastructure, support, training, and integration—when comparing build-versus-buy and vendor options.

TEFCA. The Trusted Exchange Framework and Common Agreement, a U.S. policy initiative establishing a common set of principles, terms, and technical standards to enable nationwide interoperability through participating QHINs. CPHIMS candidates should understand TEFCA's role in advancing scalable, governed health information exchange.

TOGAF. The Open Group Architecture Framework, a comprehensive methodology and toolset for developing and governing enterprise architecture, centered on the Architecture Development Method (ADM). TOGAF provides a repeatable, phased approach for aligning architecture with business strategy and managing change.

United States Core Data for Interoperability (USCDI). A standardized, regularly expanded set of health data classes and elements required for nationwide interoperable exchange under federal certification rules. USCDI defines the minimum data that certified systems must be able to share, and its versions guide interoperability planning.

User Acceptance Testing (UAT). The final validation phase in which end users confirm that a system meets business requirements and is fit for real-world use before go-live. In healthcare, UAT should mirror clinical workflows and involve frontline users to surface adoption and safety issues early.

Vendor Risk Management. The ongoing process of identifying, assessing, and mitigating risks introduced by third-party suppliers, including security, privacy, financial, and operational exposure. With heavy reliance on cloud and SaaS, healthcare leaders must conduct due diligence, require BAAs, and monitor vendors continuously.

Waterfall. A sequential, phase-gated project methodology in which each stage (requirements, design, build, test, deploy) is completed before the next begins. Waterfall offers predictability and strong documentation suited to highly regulated work but adapts poorly to changing requirements, making hybrid approaches common.

Work Breakdown Structure (WBS). A hierarchical decomposition of a project's total scope into smaller, manageable deliverables and work packages used for planning, estimating, and control. The WBS is the basis for scheduling, resource assignment, and tracking, ensuring no scope is overlooked.

Zachman Framework. An enterprise architecture ontology that classifies and organizes architectural artifacts in a matrix of perspectives (planner, owner, designer, builder, subcontractor) against interrogatives (what, how, where, who, when, why). It serves as a structured taxonomy for ensuring completeness of enterprise architecture documentation rather than a step-by-step process.

Zero-Trust. A security model based on the principle "never trust, always verify," requiring continuous authentication and authorization of every user, device, and request regardless of network location. Zero-trust architectures reduce lateral movement after a breach and are increasingly adopted in healthcare to counter ransomware and insider threats.

Governance, Architecture, and Management Frameworks Quick Reference

CPHIMS candidates are expected to recognize, distinguish, and apply a working vocabulary of governance, architecture, project, quality, security, and maturity frameworks. The exam rarely asks for a definition in isolation; instead it embeds a framework in a senior-leadership scenario and asks which one best fits the situation, or which artifact a given framework produces. The entries below give the purpose of each framework in one line so you can disambiguate them quickly under time pressure. Pay particular attention to the boundaries between frameworks that are easily confused — enterprise architecture (TOGAF vs. Zachman), IT governance vs. service management (COBIT vs. ITIL), and the family of HIMSS maturity models.

.45 Enterprise and Solution Architecture

TOGAF (The Open Group Architecture Framework). A process-oriented enterprise architecture method whose Architecture Development Method (ADM) walks an organization iteratively through architecture vision, business, information-systems (data and application), and technology architectures, then opportunities, migration planning, and governance — answering *how* to build and evolve an enterprise architecture.

Zachman Framework. A taxonomy, not a process: a 6×6 matrix that classifies architecture artifacts by interrogatives (What, How, Where, Who, When, Why) against stakeholder perspectives (Executive, Business Management, Architect, Engineer, Technician, Enterprise) — answering *what artifacts* describe an enterprise, leaving the method to frameworks like TOGAF.

.46 IT Governance and Service Management

COBIT 2019 (Control Objectives for Information and Related Technologies). ISACA's governance and management framework for enterprise information and technology, separating governance objectives (Evaluate, Direct, Monitor) from management objectives across four domains; it aligns IT to enterprise goals, defines design factors, and is the dominant reference for IT governance, risk, and control assurance.

ITIL 4 (Information Technology Infrastructure Library). A service-management framework built around the Service Value System and the four dimensions of service management, replacing ITIL v3's rigid lifecycle with 34 flexible "practices" (incident, problem, change enablement, service request, etc.) and a holistic value-stream view; it governs *how IT services are delivered and supported* day to day.

.47 Project, Program, and Portfolio Management

PMBOK / PMI (Project Management Body of Knowledge). PMI's reference standard; the 7th edition pivoted from the prior process-and-knowledge-area model to twelve principles and eight performance domains, embracing predictive, agile, and hybrid delivery — the conceptual basis for the PMP credential and the default project-management vocabulary on the exam.

PRINCE2 (PRojects IN Controlled Environments). A prescriptive, stage-gated project-management method organized around seven principles, seven themes, and seven processes with defined management products and clear governance roles (notably the Project Board); strongest where tight control, business-case justification, and accountability are required.

.48 Quality and Process Improvement

Lean. A philosophy and toolset focused on maximizing customer value while eliminating the eight wastes (defects, overproduction, waiting, non-utilized talent, transportation, inventory, motion, extra-processing —

"DOWNTIME"); in health IT it streamlines clinical and operational workflows and underpins value-stream mapping.

Six Sigma. A data-driven methodology to reduce process variation and defects toward 3.4 defects per million opportunities, executed through the DMAIC cycle (Define, Measure, Analyze, Improve, Control); frequently combined with Lean as "Lean Six Sigma" for end-to-end process-improvement programs.

.49 Performance Management

Balanced Scorecard. A strategic performance-management framework that translates strategy into measurable objectives across four perspectives — Financial, Customer, Internal Business Process, and Learning & Growth — ensuring that IT and operational metrics are linked to enterprise strategy rather than reported in isolation; often paired with strategy maps.

.50 Security and Risk Frameworks

NIST Cybersecurity Framework (CSF) 2.0. A voluntary, outcomes-based framework now organized around six functions — Govern, Identify, Protect, Detect, Respond, Recover — that helps organizations of any sector assess and improve cybersecurity posture; the 2.0 revision (2024) added the Govern function to elevate cybersecurity as an enterprise-risk discipline.

NIST AI Risk Management Framework (AI RMF 1.0). A voluntary framework structured around four functions — Govern, Map, Measure, Manage — for identifying and mitigating risks across the AI lifecycle and cultivating trustworthy, accountable AI; increasingly relevant to healthcare AI/clinical-decision-support governance and supplemented by the Generative AI Profile.

HITRUST CSF (Common Security Framework). A certifiable, prescriptive control framework that harmonizes HIPAA, NIST, ISO, PCI, and other authoritative sources into a single set of mapped controls; widely adopted by healthcare organizations and their business associates as a unifying, assessable compliance and risk-assurance standard.

ISO/IEC 27001. The international standard specifying requirements for an Information Security Management System (ISMS) — a risk-based, certifiable management system with Annex A controls and mandatory clauses for leadership, planning, support, operation, and continual improvement; the global benchmark for demonstrating systematic information-security governance.

.51 HIMSS Analytics Maturity Models

EMRAM (Electronic Medical Record Adoption Model). HIMSS Analytics' eight-stage (0–7) model that scores inpatient EMR capability and adoption, from no ancillary systems at Stage 0 through a fully paperless, advanced-analytics, closed-loop environment at Stage 7; the benchmark most candidates know best and the template for the maturity-model family.

INFRAM (Infrastructure Adoption Model). An eight-stage model assessing the maturity of the underlying technology infrastructure — mobility, security, collaboration, transport, and data-center domains — that must be in place to support advanced clinical and analytics capabilities.

DIAM and AMAM (Digital Imaging Adoption Model; Analytics Maturity Adoption Model). DIAM measures maturity of medical-imaging and image-management capability across the enterprise, while AMAM (Adoption Model for Analytics Maturity) scores an organization's progression from fragmented data toward governed, predictive, and prescriptive analytics; both extend the staged-benchmark approach beyond the core EMR.

Standards, Regulations, and Agencies Crosswalk

Interoperability and regulatory questions are a reliable share of the CPHIMS exam. The challenge is rarely deep technical detail; it is knowing which standard or rule *governs a given situation* and which body *enforces or maintains* it. This crosswalk groups the essential items by category — interoperability and data standards, privacy and security regulations, AI and data-protection law, and the U.S. programs and agencies that certify, pay for, regulate, or coordinate health IT. Learn the boundaries: HL7 v2 vs. FHIR, HIPAA Privacy vs. Security vs. Breach, ONC (certification) vs. CMS (payment and conditions), FDA (devices and SaMD).

.52 Interoperability and Data Standards

HL7 v2. The decades-old, pipe-and-hat-delimited messaging standard (e.g., ADT, ORM, ORU messages) still carrying the majority of real-time clinical transactions between systems; ubiquitous, flexible, loosely constrained, and the workhorse of intra-enterprise integration.

CDA (Clinical Document Architecture). An HL7 v3, XML-based standard for exchanging structured clinical *documents* (the Consolidated CDA / C-CDA templates underlie the Continuity of Care Document and transition-of-care summaries); document-centric, in contrast to FHIR's resource-and-API model.

FHIR R4 (Fast Healthcare Interoperability Resources, Release 4). HL7's modern, web/REST-based standard that models clinical and administrative concepts as modular "resources" exchanged via APIs (often with the SMART on FHIR app-launch and OAuth2 authorization layer); R4 is the first normative release and the foundation of U.S. certified API requirements.

USCDI (United States Core Data for Interoperability). ONC's standardized set of health-data classes and elements (demographics, problems, medications, lab results, clinical notes, and expanding versions) that all certified systems must be able to exchange; it defines the minimum *content* floor that FHIR and C-CDA must carry.

IHE (Integrating the Healthcare Enterprise). Not a standard but an initiative that publishes *integration profiles* (e.g., XDS for document sharing, PIX/PDQ for patient identity, ATNA for audit/security) specifying how to combine existing standards like HL7, DICOM, and FHIR to solve concrete interoperability use cases.

DICOM (Digital Imaging and Communications in Medicine). The universal standard for storing, transmitting, and managing medical images and associated metadata; governs PACS, modality communication, and image objects across radiology, cardiology, and other imaging-intensive specialties.

X12 (ASC X12). The EDI standard family governing administrative and financial transactions mandated under HIPAA — eligibility (270/271), claims (837), remittance (835), claim status (276/277), and enrollment — the backbone of revenue-cycle and payer–provider data exchange.

.53 Privacy and Security Regulations

HIPAA Privacy Rule. Establishes national standards for the use and disclosure of Protected Health Information (PHI), defines individual rights (access, amendment, accounting of disclosures), the minimum-necessary standard, and permitted disclosures for treatment, payment, and operations; governs *who may see and share* PHI.

HIPAA Security Rule. Sets requirements for safeguarding electronic PHI (ePHI) through administrative, physical, and technical safeguards — risk analysis, access controls, audit controls, transmission security, and the like — and is the rule most directly tied to a health-IT leader's day-to-day controls.

HIPAA Breach Notification Rule. Requires covered entities and business associates to notify affected individuals, HHS, and (for large breaches) the media following a breach of unsecured PHI, with timelines and risk-assessment criteria for determining when notification is triggered.

HITECH Act (Health Information Technology for Economic and Clinical Health). The 2009 law that funded EHR adoption (Meaningful Use), strengthened HIPAA enforcement and penalties, extended direct liability to business associates, and created the breach-notification mandate; the legislative engine behind a generation of health-IT modernization.

21st Century Cures Act and the Information Blocking Rule. The 2016 Cures Act and ONC's implementing rule prohibit "information blocking" — practices that unreasonably interfere with access, exchange, or use of electronic health information — by providers, developers of certified health IT, and HIEs/HINs, subject to defined exceptions; it also mandated standardized FHIR-based API access for patients.

.54 AI and Data-Protection Law

EU AI Act. The European Union's risk-tiered regulation of artificial intelligence (entering into force in 2024 with phased application through 2026 and beyond) that classifies AI systems as unacceptable, high, limited, or minimal risk and imposes conformity, transparency, and governance obligations; many clinical-AI and medical-device AI systems fall in the high-risk tier, making it relevant to global health-IT strategy.

GDPR (General Data Protection Regulation). The EU's comprehensive data-protection law governing the processing of personal data, with principles of lawfulness, purpose limitation, data minimization, and accountability, strong data-subject rights, breach-notification duties, and substantial fines; the global reference point for privacy and a frequent contrast case to HIPAA.

.55 U.S. Programs, Certification, and Agencies

ONC Health IT Certification Program. The Assistant Secretary for Technology Policy / Office of the National Coordinator program (operating under the ONC Certification Criteria, including the Cures Act "Health IT Certification Program" updates) that tests and certifies health IT to required capabilities — USCDI support, FHIR-based APIs, security, and information-blocking compliance — so that certified products qualify for federal programs.

CMS Promoting Interoperability Programs. The Centers for Medicare & Medicaid Services programs (successors to Meaningful Use) that tie Medicare/Medicaid incentives and penalties to eligible hospitals' and clinicians' use of certified EHR technology, reporting on measures such as electronic prescribing, health-information exchange, and public-health reporting.

CMS Conditions of Participation (CoPs). The federal health-and-safety requirements hospitals and other providers must meet to participate in Medicare and Medicaid; relevant to health IT through requirements such as electronic notifications of admission/discharge/transfer (the patient-event notification CoP) and medical-record and QAPI standards.

FDA Software as a Medical Device (SaMD). The Food and Drug Administration's framework (aligned with IMDRF guidance) for regulating software that performs a medical function independent of hardware, including risk-based classification, premarket pathways, and evolving guidance on AI/ML-enabled devices and predetermined change-control plans; it determines when clinical software is a regulated device.

TEFCA and the RCE (Trusted Exchange Framework and Common Agreement; Recognized Coordinating Entity). TEFCA establishes a national "network of networks" floor for interoperability; the Common Agreement is the legal/technical contract that Qualified Health Information Networks (QHINs) sign, and the RCE (operated by The Sequoia Project) administers and enforces it — the framework for nationwide, governed exchange.

HHS 405(d) Program. The Department of Health and Human Services cybersecurity program established under the Cybersecurity Act of 2015 Section 405(d), which publishes the *Health Industry Cybersecurity Practices (HICP)* — voluntary, consensus-based practices addressing the top threats to the sector — and aligns to the Health Care and Public Health (HPH) Cybersecurity Performance Goals.

Exam-Day Strategy and the Two-Week Final Review

The CPHIMS examination tests the judgment of a senior health-IT leader, not the recall of a technician. Most stems are multi-sentence scenarios that place you in a management role and ask for the *best*, *first*, or *most appropriate* action. Success depends as much on disciplined test-taking as on content mastery. This appendix gives you concrete tactics for the computer-based exam and a structured fourteen-day review plan keyed to the domains of this guide.

.56 Knowing the Exam Format

The CPHIMS is a computer-based, multiple-choice examination delivered at testing centers and via remote proctoring. It comprises 115 items, of which 100 are scored and 15 are unscored pretest items seeded throughout — you cannot tell which is which, so treat every question as if it counts. You have two hours of testing time. That works out to just over one minute per item on average, which is comfortable *if* you do not let a handful of hard scenarios drain the clock. Scoring is scaled; there is no penalty for guessing beyond a wrong answer, so never leave an item blank.

.57 Time and Clock Management

Budget in three passes. Plan for roughly 75 to 80 minutes on a first pass through all items, leaving the remainder for a second pass on flagged questions and a final pass to confirm nothing is unanswered. At the two-hour total, aim to finish the first pass with at least 35 to 40 minutes in reserve.

Set checkpoints. Glance at the on-screen timer at fixed marks — for example, you should be near item 30 at the 35-minute mark and near item 60 at the 70-minute mark. If you fall behind, you are dwelling too long; start flagging and moving.

Flag and move; never stall. The moment a question makes you reread the stem a third time, choose your best provisional answer, flag it for review, and advance. A question you stare at for four minutes costs you the chance to bank two or three easy ones later. The review screen lets you return to every flagged item.

Answer everything before the final flag-clear. In your last pass, make sure no item is unanswered. An educated guess beats a blank every time because there is no negative marking.

.58 Reading Senior-Scenario Stems

Identify your role and your scope. Most stems cast you as a CIO, director of health informatics, project sponsor, or governance-committee chair. The correct answer is the one appropriate to *that* level of authority — a senior leader convenes a steering committee, commissions a risk analysis, or escalates to governance; a senior leader does not personally re-cable a switch or write the SQL.

Find the actual question. Read the *last* sentence first when a stem is long. The call-to-action ("Which action should the CIO take *first*?") tells you what kind of answer to hunt for and lets you read the body purposefully rather than passively.

Underline (mentally) the constraints. Scenarios bury decisive qualifiers: a regulatory deadline, a fixed budget, a stated patient-safety risk, an in-flight project, a union or board dynamic. The constraint usually eliminates two distractors immediately.

Watch for the embedded framework. When a stem mentions an EMRAM stage, a risk analysis, an information-blocking complaint, or a change-control failure, it is signaling which body of knowledge the answer lives in. Map the scenario to the framework before you read the options.

.59 Eliminating Distractors

Cross out the technically-correct-but-wrong-scope option. A frequent trap pairs a valid technical action with a question whose correct answer is a *governance or process* step. The technical action is real, even attractive, but premature given the leader's role.

Reject absolutes and "do nothing." Options containing *always*, *never*, *only*, or *immediately terminate* are usually wrong in a profession built on risk-based judgment. Likewise, "take no action" is rarely correct unless the stem establishes that intervention would violate a rule.

Beware the unprioritized-correct option. In *BEST/FIRST* questions, two or three options may all be things you *would* do — but only one is what you do *first* or *best*. Eliminating the obviously wrong answers is only half the job; you must then sequence the survivors.

Use the "would I be criticized?" test. Imagine defending each remaining option to a board or auditor. The choice that survives scrutiny — the one a prudent leader could justify — is almost always correct.

.60 Handling "BEST," "FIRST," and "MOST APPROPRIATE"

These qualifiers are the signature of the CPHIMS, and they have a reliable logic:

FIRST = sequence. The question asks what comes earliest in a correct chain of actions. The right answer is usually the *assessment, analysis, or stakeholder-engagement* step that must precede execution. Before you fix, you scope; before you scope, you assess. A risk analysis precedes selecting a control; requirements precede a vendor selection.

BEST = optimization among valid options. Several options work; one optimizes for the stem's stated priority (patient safety, compliance, cost, sustainability). Re-read the constraint and pick the option that maximizes *that* value.

MOST APPROPRIATE = role and context fit. The answer must match the leader's authority, the organization's maturity, and the regulatory context. An action that is appropriate for a mature, well-resourced system may be inappropriate for the one described.

The governance-step vs. technical-step rule. When in doubt between a process answer (charter a committee, conduct a risk assessment, follow change management, escalate to governance, engage stakeholders) and a technical answer (apply a patch, reconfigure the firewall, migrate the database), the senior-scenario framing usually favors the *governance or process* step — unless the stem establishes an active, time-critical technical emergency (a live outage, an in-progress breach) where immediate containment is the correct *first* action. Match the answer to the urgency and to your role.

.61 The Two-Week Final Review Plan

This fourteen-day plan assumes your substantive study is largely complete and you are in consolidation mode. It is keyed to the guide's domains and balances content review, practice testing, and rest. Adjust the daily hours to your schedule, but keep the rhythm: review, then test, then remediate.

Day 1 — Diagnostic baseline. Take a full-length, timed practice exam under realistic conditions (two hours, no interruptions). Score it, then categorize every miss by domain. This diagnostic, not your gut feeling, sets your priorities for the next twelve days.

Day 2 — General Knowledge of Healthcare and Technology Environments. Review healthcare delivery models, organizational structures, reimbursement, regulatory bodies, and the technology landscape. Re-read Appendix E's agencies and programs section. Do 25 to 30 domain-targeted practice items.

Day 3 — Systems Analysis and Design (part 1). Review requirements gathering, workflow analysis, process mapping, and the systems development life cycle. Practice translating a clinical workflow problem into requirements. 25 items.

Day 4 — Systems Analysis and Design (part 2). Review interoperability standards in depth — re-read Appendix E's standards section and be able to distinguish HL7 v2, C-CDA, FHIR R4, USCDI, IHE, DICOM, and X12 on sight. 25 items focused on standards selection.

Day 5 — Systems Selection, Implementation, Support, and Maintenance. Review vendor selection, RFP processes, contract considerations, go-live planning, training, and lifecycle support. Reinforce ITIL 4 practices and change management from Appendix D. 25 items.

Day 6 — Mid-point full practice exam. Take a second timed, full-length exam. Compare your domain scores against the Day 1 diagnostic to confirm your weak areas are improving and to surface any new gaps. Categorize misses.

Day 7 — Administration and Leadership (part 1). Review strategic planning, governance structures, IT steering committees, and aligning IT to organizational strategy. Reinforce COBIT 2019, TOGAF, and the Balanced Scorecard from Appendix D. 25 items.

Day 8 — Administration and Leadership (part 2). Review financial management, budgeting, capital vs. operating expense, total cost of ownership, ROI, staffing, and human-resource considerations. Practice the financial-priority *BEST* questions. 25 items.

Day 9 — Privacy and Security (part 1). Review the HIPAA Privacy, Security, and Breach Notification Rules and HITECH in depth from Appendix E. Drill the administrative, physical, and technical safeguards. 25 security-domain items.

Day 10 — Privacy and Security (part 2) and Risk. Review the NIST CSF 2.0 functions, NIST AI RMF, HITRUST, ISO 27001, and HHS 405(d) HICP from Appendices D and E. Practice risk-analysis-as-first-step scenarios. 25 items.

Day 11 — Project Management and weakest domain. Review PMBOK principles, PRINCE2, and Lean/Six Sigma from Appendix D. Then spend the remaining time on whichever single domain your two practice exams show as weakest. 25 to 30 mixed items.

Day 12 — Third full practice exam. Take a final timed, full-length exam. Your goal is a comfortable margin above passing across all domains. Categorize misses one last time, but resist cramming new material — this late, refinement beats expansion.

Day 13 — Targeted remediation and tactics rehearsal. Work only the specific item types and topics you are still missing. Re-read the "Reading Senior-Scenario Stems," "Eliminating Distractors," and "BEST/FIRST/MOST APPROPRIATE" sections above and consciously apply each tactic to ten practice scenarios. Confirm exam logistics: location or remote-proctor setup, identification, scheduled time, and system check.

Day 14 — Light review and rest. Do no more than a light skim of Appendices D and E and your personal cheat sheet of confused-pairs (TOGAF vs. Zachman, COBIT vs. ITIL, Privacy vs. Security Rule, ONC vs. CMS vs. FDA, FIRST vs. BEST). Stop studying by early afternoon. Sleep is a performance variable; protect it. Arrive early, breathe, and trust your preparation.

.62 Final Reminders

Read every option before choosing, even when the first looks right — the CPHIMS rewards the *best* answer, and a better one often sits in position C or D. Trust your first instinct on changes: only alter an answer when you find a concrete reason in the stem, not on a vague feeling. Keep your role and scope in mind on every scenario. And manage the clock so that the last forty minutes belong to you, not to two questions that ran away with the hour.

www.ingramcontent.com/pod-product-compliance
Lightning Source LLC
LaVergne TN
LVHW062028051126
851858LV00005B/114